Prescription for Maximum Savings

Jason Reed PharmD

Copyright © 2018 Jason Reed

All rights reserved.

ISBN-13:978-1-7312-8442-6

The information provided in this book is designed to help you have a conversation with your doctor and healthcare team about your medications. It is not intended as a substitute for any treatment that may have been prescribed by your doctor. You should always discuss changes in your medication regimen with your doctor prior to making them.

CONTENTS

	Acknowledgments	i
1	Introduction	Pg 1
2	Chapter 1: Medication Facts & Figures	Pg 6
3	Chapter 2: Why do Drugs Cost so Much?	Pg 9
4	Chapter 3: Where Have We Been and Where Are We Headed?	Pg 18
5	Chapter 4: Insurance Mumbo Jumbo	Pg 22
6	Step 1: Medication List	Pg 24
7	Step 2: Drug Discontinuation	Pg 32
8	Step 3: Journaling	Pg 38
9	Step 4: Schedule a Medication Review	Pg 40
10	Step 5: Got Vaccines?	Pg 42
11	Step 6: Lifestyle Changes	Pg 44
12	Step 7: How Do I Save Using My Insurance	Pg 48
13	Step 8: Are You A Veteran?	Pg 52
14	Step 9: Could It be Cheaper to Pay Cash?	Pg 54
15	Step 10: Drug Discount Programs	Pg 56
16	Step 11: Generics	Pg 59
17	Step 12: Therapeutic Equivalents	Pg 62
18	Step 13: Pharmacy Types	Pg 67
19	Step 14: Check the Quantity	Pg 72
20	Step 15: Tablet Splitting	Pg 74

21	Step 16: Combo Pills	Pg 76
22	Step 17: Dosage Forms	Pg 78
23	Step 18: Review Your Allergies and Intolerances	Pg 82
24	Step 19: Samples	Pg 84
25	Step 20: Pharmaceutical Assistance Programs (PAP's)	Pg 86
26	Step 21: State Pharmaceutical Assistance Programs	Pg 93
27	Step 22: Pharmaceutical Manufacturer Copay Coupons	Pg 95
28	Step 23: Expiration Dates	Pg 99
29	Step 24: Specialty Pharmacy and Biosimilars	Pg101
30	Step 25: Keeping it All Straight – Technology Tools	Pg107
31	Step 26: Repeat This Process Each Year!	Pg109
32	Final Thoughts	Pg113
33	Appendix A – Terminology	Pg115
34	Appendix B – Medication List	Pg120
35	Appendix C – Medication Talking Points	Pg123
36	About the Author	Pg128
37	References	Pg129

Jason Reed

Prescription for Maximum Savings

Jason Reed

ACKNOWLEDGMENTS

I am grateful to the many people who contributed to the completion of this book. I extend a heartfelt thank you to all the family, friends and colleagues who supported me in what was a very large undertaking.

I would like to thank Shawnn Welde, my editor. She spent many hours poring through the pharmacist speak and translating into something that is reader friendly. I appreciate your editing expertise.

Finally, to my wife and kids who put up with me during this process and supported me all the way.

Introduction

You found this book because you know that medication is overpriced. You probably also know medication is extremely overprescribed. According to a study published in *JAMA: The Journal of the American Medical Association*, the per capita spending on prescription drugs in the US is higher than in all other industrialized nations.[1] Recent news headlines have played into the fear and anger generated by this massive overspending. Examples include "Prescription Price Crisis," "Prescription Drug Costs in the US are a Crime," "How an $84,000 Drug Got Its Price," and "Outcry on EpiPen Prices Hasn't Made Them Lower." After you read the articles pointing fingers at the various players, one problem remains. How do you protect yourself from high prices and too much medicine?

Cost shifting from payers and employers to patients has been the trend in recent years and is predicted to accelerate. More Americans are concerned about health care costs (85%) than are concerned about retirement (73%), housing (66%), and child care (49%), according to a recent survey.[2] High deductibles, more copay tiers, and very high out of pocket maximums impact patients' wallets directly. Medical bills are a leading cause of bankruptcy in the U.S. The only thing that leads to higher bills than the cost of taking medications as prescribed is not taking them. When patients can't afford to take the medication as prescribed, they all too often wind up in the most expensive part of the healthcare system... the emergency room.

The problem is multifaceted, and there is plenty of blame to go around. Pharmaceutical companies, insurance middlemen, large health systems and government programs all play a part in the steep increase in a patient's out of pocket costs. In addition, advancements in pharmaceutical treatments and biologic therapies are rapidly evolving, adding to the higher costs. This book will review the drivers behind these problems and the developing trends that will affect the money spent on medications and healthcare in the future.

In this book, I am going to show you how to save money and eliminate unneeded medication use. A step-by-step process for reviewing your medication list, insurance, cash pay and over the counter options will enable you to maximize your savings on your healthcare dollars. No one solution will work for all patients, which is why having a system to ensure you don't miss out on any of the savings opportunities is a must. Patients must take charge of their healthcare and act like consumers, much as you do when shopping for a bike on Amazon or at a retail store. Armed with the knowledge of the costs of the products you are going to purchase leads you to the next step. Developing a relationship with your prescriber and pharmacist that is cooperative and has open communication channels is a major key to saving money on medication. Just like any successful endeavor, you need a carefully built team of healthcare professionals around you to help you achieve maximum health and wellness for your body and wallet. This book will give you a holistic approach to obtaining the correct medications at the lowest cost to you; not just by finding the lowest prices on medications, but also by helping you find the best type of insurance that makes the most sense given the medication regimen you may have.

As a practicing pharmacist for over 15 years, I have seen the amount patients pay out of pocket climb over the years. I worked for a large pharmacy benefits manager and worked closely with health insurers as benefit setups evolved over time. I have also spent time working around prior authorization processes on the side of both the prescriber and the payer. Most recently, I have worked to provide more pricing and benefit information to prescribers, so they can relay the information to the patient at the point of care while the patient is still in the office. I was inspired to write this book while sitting in a meeting with many healthcare professionals and executives from various healthcare companies. It was clear to me that very few of the people in that meeting really understood how prescription benefits worked. I thought to myself, if these people don't understand, then how can the average patient. I started thinking back to all the friends and family who, over the years, had asked me questions about the rising cost of their medications. Light bulb! Why not create a resource for patients to use? I could sift through all the noise and get down to the core savings techniques. With my diverse background and experiences in pharmacy benefits and my clinical knowledge as a pharmacist, I could share my knowledge of cost savings with as many patients as possible.

I have had to put these practices into place for my own family. A transition from one employer to another in my career also meant a transition to a new insurance company and new prescription drug coverage as well. Each time a change occurred, I had to work through a web of determining questions. Will my scripts be covered? Can I still use my local pharmacy that I know and trust? Does it make sense to use mail order?

During the last open enrollment, I was able to save $600 annually for a family member who was using just two prescriptions. Unfortunately, prescribers are busy, and the office staff often are not well versed on how to save patients money on their medications. In addition, not everyone has a pharmacist in the family who can take the time to look in depth at their medications. The most useful resource for a patient, the community pharmacist, is often strapped for time trying to dispense prescriptions and does not have the time for an in-depth discussion on how to save money on prescriptions.

This book will show you how to use the resources that are available to you, so you spend less on your medications. Spending less leads to a higher likelihood that the medication will be used as prescribed. This in turn will lower out of pocket costs for other medical problems that arise from not using medication as prescribed. In addition, the reduced financial burden will lessen stress and lead to better outcomes. Finally, don't think of this as a onetime read, but as a resource that you will return to again and again. Each year as your medical coverage changes, pull out this book and look at where you fall in the step-by-step process based on your plan for the upcoming year. The great news for living today is medical breakthroughs happen every day and will continue to happen. That means you will eventually end up needing some type of medication to support you in your longer life expectancy. Knowing how to maximize savings will be key. The centenarian (people who are 100 years or older) population has exploded. According to Centers for Disease Control and Prevention, in 2014 there were 72,197 centenarians, which is up 44 percent since the year 2000. Most of the people in this age group take five or more prescription medications. Will you be prepared to maximize savings as a longer life inevitably leads to disease states that you may need to control with medication?

Many blog posts and websites out there claim to be able to save you money. If you can find this information on the internet, why do you need this book? The answer is simple: too many options and too many things to do or investigate. How can you keep it all straight? How will you know when you have maximized your savings options? Who can help you navigate the vast array of discount offers? Without a plan, you will end up with disappointing results and feel helpless. That is exactly why you need this book, to guide you step by step on how to maximize every available opportunity.

The benefit tips and tricks you are about to read have proven results. Each chapter provides new secrets that will help you stay in control of your medication costs. Don't wait to realize these types of rewards for yourself. I can promise you the stepwise approach will save you money. Most will save hundreds per year and many can save thousands depending on how many medications you take. If you follow the formula in this book you will very likely cut your out of pocket expenses by up to 50% and in some cases by much more.

   This stepwise approach saved a schoolteacher $759 per year by adjusting the number of refills she was getting on her asthma inhalers. She did not realize she should only use the rescue inhaler as needed for immediate relief from acute attacks, and she was noncompliant with using the steroid inhaler she was supposed to use daily. Not only did she save money on her prescriptions, but because she was now in compliance, she also cut down on her many trips to the ER, an even greater benefit that probably saved her thousands.

   One patient who was 68 years old was able to save $432 per year by reviewing her medication list and eliminating a drug she no longer needed. She was given a medication to help her sleep after a hospital admission. The medication was never discontinued; as often happens, at her follow up appointment, another sleep aid was prescribed because the prescriber didn't realize she was already taking one. Aside from eliminating an unneeded cost, the biggest savings was preventing excessive drowsiness that could have led to her falling and landing right back in the hospital.

   Another younger patient was able to consolidate his blood pressure medications into a combination pill that saved him $250 annually and improved his compliance. The refills for the two previously prescribed medications were staggered, and he would often run out of one or the other, never truly taking both together.

   A patient recently diagnosed with MS was able to save $2500 per year by looking at the formulary options her insurance preferred. She found an MS medication that had a biosimilar on the formulary, and she asked her doctor to prescribe that medication. She was able to lower her insurance copay and increased her savings with a manufacturer coupon. Had she not realized those savings, it is likely that private school for her son or the next family vacation would have been on the chopping block.

   I could go on and on with examples of how savings have been realized by putting this system in place. All too often, people just take the high prices the pharmacist tells them at the counter as gospel, deciding later it was too expensive. This leads to the second fill not being picked up, and that is not an effective process for anyone. Let's get started on minimizing your drug costs RIGHT NOW! I call you to act and become a proactive consumer of your own healthcare needs. Let's help bring drug spending in line, one patient at a time.

Regarding pricing shown in this book. All are cash prices from GoodRx (see Step 10) prices are subject to change at any time and vary greatly by location and other factors.

.

Chapter 1   Medication Facts and Figures

The United States is spending almost twice as much as other developed countries on healthcare 3.3 trillion, or 17.9% of gross domestic product in 2016.[3] From 2007 to 2014, middle class families increased spending on health care by almost 25%. As shown in figure 1 below, while the spending on healthcare increased, spending on other basic needs decreased.[4]

Figure 1

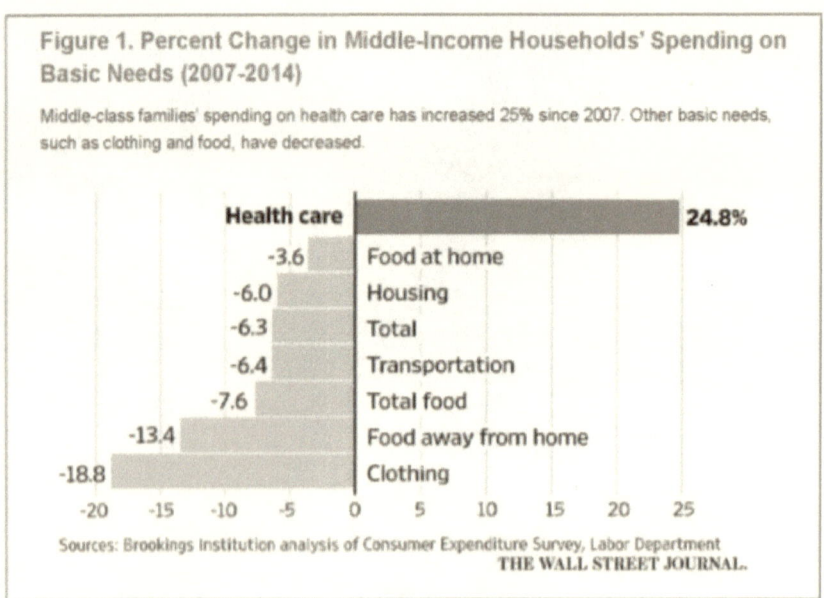

Despite raises in wages, the net take home pay did not actually increase because of the skyrocketing cost of health care premiums and deductibles. Premiums increased 20% since 2011 while deductibles increased 49% over the same period.[5] This kind of cost inflation puts a drag on the economy. With less money going back into the economy, employers can't hire as many workers, and too many families, struggling to make ends meet, must choose between basic needs or health coverage.

The number of prescriptions filled for Americans, both adults and children, rose 85 percent between 1997 and 2016 from 2.4 billion to 4.5 billion a year, while the U.S. population rose only 21 percent according to the health research firm Quintile IMS.[6] These facts coupled with the data from a new survey find that 55 percent of Americans regularly take a prescription medicine -- and they're taking more than ever.[7] A survey done by Consumer Reports shows that those who use prescription drugs take, on average, FOUR prescriptions, and many also take over-the-counter drugs, vitamins and other dietary supplements. Many of the prescriptions taken are unneeded and often prescribed to control harmful side effects from other prescription medications. To make matters worse, some get medications not prescribed by a clinician.

Among those who take prescription drugs, 53 percent get them from more than one health care provider. This often leads to miscommunication or no communication between prescribers and greatly increases the likelihood of adverse drug effects. More than a third of people surveyed say no provider has reviewed their medicines to see if all are necessary. In 2014, nearly 1.3 million people sought emergency room treatment for adverse drug effects, and about 124,000 people died, according to U.S. government data cited by Consumer Reports.

The good news...medication is helping to increase life expectancy, and quality of life in the latter decades is at a place it has never been before. Modern medicine has cured many crippling diseases already and will continue to do so in the future.

The bad news... medication costs can be extreme and have increased substantially over other goods and services. Bankruptcy due to medical bills was a central argument during the battle over the passage of Obamacare. Certainly, some specialty medications could leave patients in a financial crisis. When a new health problem is diagnosed, often the patient's income declines, reeking financial havoc on that patient's family. The financial worries coupled with the stress of their newly found health problem are bound to lead to worse outcomes from the ailment.

Waiting for the folks in Washington to fix the problems of your healthcare costs is not an effective game plan. Stepping up and acting to control your costs now and in the future is vital. You need to consider your healthcare options in the same way you would consider booking a trip online. Start by comparison shopping and researching all your options to find the best overall value. By picking up this book, you are on the right path. You have taken the first step. Once you read this book and discover savings for yourself, the next step would be to act by passing it along to a friend or family member. Remember, reports state that one in four patients in California report that they did not get their script filled due to cost concerns.[8] Could one of those folks be your friend or family member? Does simply not getting the script filled sound like the most effective way to control healthcare costs for that patient? Not filling the script could result in them being unable to work due to problems with their disease state. Please do your part and help me spread the word on this mounting crisis in healthcare. We all need to do our part to help bring this back under control.

Chapter 2 Why Do Drugs Cost So Much?

As I thought about how to explain this very complex subject in an easily digestible manner, it dawned on me that most people blame drug companies for high drug prices. Let me assure you that there is plenty of blame to go around, and not all of it is big Pharma. Many pitfalls exist in our current system of pricing and payment for both health insurance and prescription medications. Please take a few minutes to read the background that will help you understand why you need to follow my step-by-step process.

Many people may ask, "Does it really cost that much for a pharmaceutical manufacturer to take some basic chemicals and mix them together into a medication that helps with my high blood pressure?" It is a great question, and on the surface, it does in fact look like it should be that simple. What most people don't understand is that for every drug that makes it to the market for human consumption, there are between 3,000-5,000 compounds that fail along the path and are never able to be sold.

A drug is not suddenly discovered and then ready to go on the shelves at your local pharmacy. In the United States, the Food and Drug Administration (FDA) has a rigorous process that entails five phases of testing that must be done to bring a drug to market. It takes many different drug products through various phases of testing to find the one that makes it. In many cases, it can take 12 to 15 years for a drug to be approved by the FDA under what is called an NDA (New Drug Application). The FDA confirms whether the drug is safe and effective for its proposed uses and whether the benefits of the drug outweigh the risks. The FDA never considers price when looking to approve a drug, only the safety and efficacy. This will be important to remember later when we discuss drug prices.

Figure 2

The Drug Development process in the U.S.
Phase 1: Discovery and Development
Phase 2: Preclinical Research
Phase 3: Clinical Research
Phase 4: FDA Drug Review
Phase 5: FDA Post-Market Drug Safety Monitoring

Each of the steps listed in the table can take from a few months to several years and cost millions of dollars. Clinical research testing alone can take multiple years because of the different stages involved in the trials. The testing begins first in animals and then proceeds to healthy humans. The final stage of testing targets humans with the disease the drug is supposed to treat. All testing must be completed before the FDA even begins to review the drug in step 4. Please note in Step 5 that although the FDA continues to monitor the drug after its approval, they are only considering the safety of the product in the general patient population. They are no longer monitoring the drug to make sure it is still effective at treating the disease.

Why do drug companies charge so much? When a drug company creates a molecule (the actual drug before it has a name), they file for a patent that is typically good for 20 years. When the patent expires, other manufacturers come in and start making generic versions, greatly decreasing the number of patients who still take the original brand drug under which the patent was filed. If it takes 12 of the 20 years to get the drug approved, no profits can be made until year 12 of the patent, leaving only 8 years to make a profit. Oh, and don't forget the other 3000-5000 molecules that had patents too but never made it through the process because they caused cancer in test mice or had some other issue. Those will never be able to become profitable for the drug company. I think you can see that a drug company must make its money while it can in order to stay profitable. However, they are not off the hook for the prices they set either.

All the years of research and development are driven in part by the FDA requiring a manufacturer in the U.S. to comply with its guidelines to be able to sell in our market. The rest of the world does not have such stringent guidelines for testing of safety and efficacy. In addition, there are many benefits gained by the rest of the world for the R&D put into by manufacturers in the U.S. Recently there has been talk that other countries who participate in the scientific advances made by large companies in the U.S. should have to pay into the system to help bring prices down overall. Stay tuned to see what comes out of these ideas.

Some drug companies will do things to extend the life of the patent. Common examples are coming up with a new dosage form, think Wellbutrin vs Wellbutrin SR vs Wellbutrin XL. Original Wellbutrin had a short half-life and was dosed three times per day. Then Wellbutrin SR was introduced which had a longer half-life and could be dosed twice per day. Finally, Wellbutrin XL was released. It had an even longer half-life and could be dosed once per day. The change in the formula made it easier for the patient to take, but each change also extended the brand life for the manufacturer, making it easier for them to keep the profits rolling in on the more expensive brand product. Another example of patent life extension came from Celexa. Two years before it was to lose its patent, the manufacturer, Forest Laboratories, won FDA approval for Lexapro, which was the same compound but had a purified version of Celexa's molecular structure. The differences in outcomes for patients with depression were never shown to be significant, but the cost they paid at the pharmacy was very different from the generic Celexa.

Media headlines have called out drug companies for price gouging. An article in the New York Times reported that New York State officials demanded that Vertex Pharmaceuticals lower the prices on their cystic fibrosis drug, Orkambi, which costs $272,000 per year. Found to be only moderately more effective than the current therapies, New York State is demanding a price reduction from the manufacturer for its Medicaid patients because the new drug is "not worth the price." This goes back to the problem I referenced earlier. The FDA only looks at safety and efficacy of a drug vs placebo (sugar pill) and has no concept of the relative price of the therapy.

Generic manufacturers have been part of the problem as well. Turing Pharmaceuticals recently raised the prices of a rarely used medication,

Daraprim, a medication used for infections, more than 550% from $13.50 to $750 per tablet. According to the New York Times article, the drug has been available for 62 years, well past any patent life.[9] The scariest part of this story was that once the media called out Turing, the CEO came out and defended the price increase, stating that other newer therapies that can save your life cost much more.

Direct to consumer advertising, which has done nothing but grow in frequency over time, (See figure 3 below from Statista through 2018[10]) is another driver of increased cost, causing greater utilization of these high-priced drugs. Drug companies spend not millions, but billions on advertising to the consumer for a drug that is often the same or only nominally better than a lower cost therapeutic alternative. However, the ad makes it sound like the drug will cure the disease in many cases.

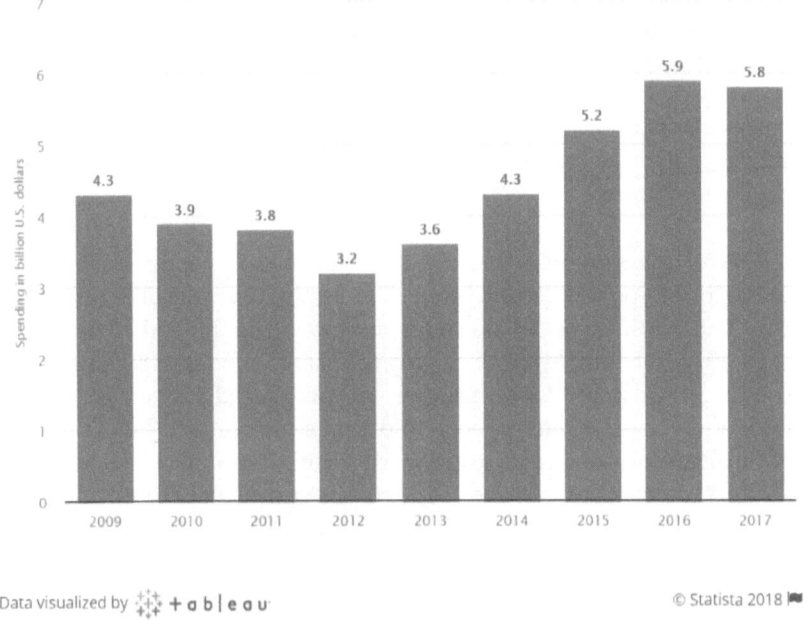

Figure 3

Even though the FDA requires the manufacturers to list all the side effects of the drug in their advertisement, the overall visual depiction is of everyone having a wonderful experience and clear improvement from using the drug. The consumer does not see the sticker shock at the pharmacy register or the adverse effects that can often occur. Today, many patients walk into their doctor's office armed with a diagnosis they found online and a medication they think they need because they saw a commercial, their minds made up before even talking to the prescriber. Some lawmakers have talked of making drug companies include the price in their ads; something that I think would be very eye opening for much of the population.

Another driver of costs is government regulation. The FDA oversees the processes to bring a drug to market. This includes testing via a new drug application mentioned above, but also includes rigorous good manufacturing practices (GMP). What is that you ask? GMP is a system for ensuring products are produced according to certain quality standards. GMP is designed to keep patients safe from inadvertent problems from the potent chemicals used to make pharmaceuticals. While this process is certainly important, in recent years it has caused prices of medications, including generics, to increase, and, in some cases, caused a critical shortage of vital life sustaining medications. The margins on generic drugs are thin, and when new GMP rules are implemented or violations identified, it drives generic drug makers out of a certain product. When this happens, it eliminates competition and drives prices up. In some extreme cases, it has caused the only maker of a drug to have to shut down operations, making the product completely unavailable.

No discussion on high costs would be complete without talking about the insurance middlemen, referred to as pharmacy benefits managers (PBM). These companies administer a pharmacy benefit for the insurer, which is often your employer. They pay the claims submitted by the pharmacies, institute the formularies, set up copays, and institute processes for prior authorization when needed to obtain a medication. Pharmacy benefit managers work directly with pharmaceutical manufacturers and drug wholesalers to negotiate prices, so your employer doesn't have to do this step. They also may own retail and or mail order pharmacies and large-scale specialty pharmacies. Being so integrated into the entire distributions system makes them ripe for conflicts of interest. Congress for many years now has been calling for more transparency around PBM's. They have been putting up spectacular numbers on Wall Street, with few people truly understanding how they make their money. The system is complex, but the larger problem boils down to the rebates they obtain from pharmaceutical manufacturers. The drug companies want to have their high-priced drug on the PBM's formulary to drive more market share. The more market share the PBM can give the manufacturer the more rebates the manufacturer will give the PBM. The misaligned incentives are that, instead of the PBM wanting the lowest cost drug in a class to be used, they will allow drug on their formulary to be prescribed without question even though it is higher priced. The PBM will get a bigger rebate than if the low-cost therapeutic option is selected. If you are a patient that can mean the difference in a copay or deductible payment of $20 vs $200. So, if the list price is high, but the pharmaceutical manufacturer gives the PBM a big rebate and then gives the patient financial assistance with their copay, who is really making out on the deal? See the below simplified version of a diagram from economist and blogger Adam Fein that shows the complexities of how drugs move through the distribution channel in the U.S.[11]

Figure 4

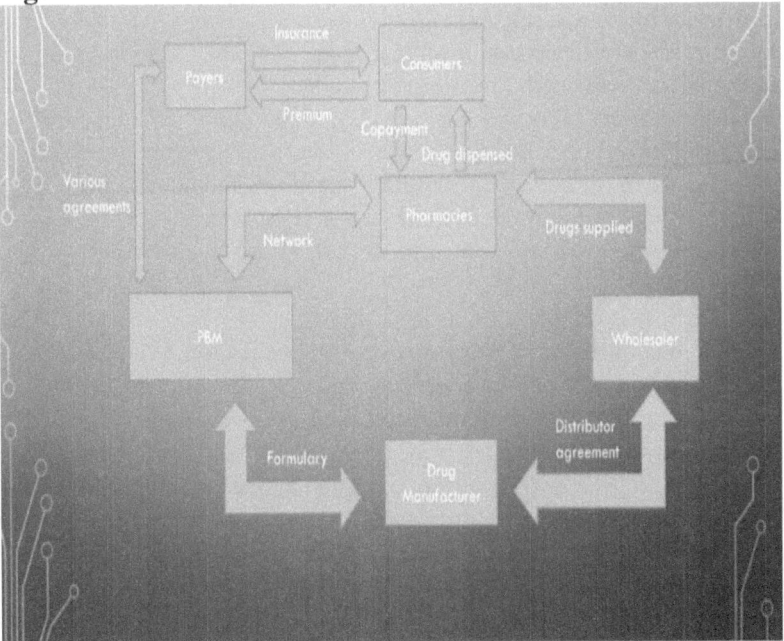

That directly leads to the next problem on the list. When your doctor prescribes a medication for you, do you ask how much it will cost? If not, why? Are you intimidated by your prescriber as many people are? Many times, the prescriber doesn't know how much the medication costs, and most would allow a different product to be used if they knew a lower cost option was available. Remember your prescriber is bombarded with things to remember. They must know in depth details of diagnosis, imaging, labs, procedures, disease pathology and on and on. A typical prescriber in med school has only had about 2 semesters of classes on medications themselves. None of that contained information about how much drugs cost. Rather your doctor was trying to learn about a product or two from each medication class to treat a disease state. At the end of the day, your prescriber wants you to use the meds he/she prescribes, but if the medication is cost-prohibitive, they can find a cheaper alternative for you in most cases. Do you think they won't have time for that? Well they may indeed be very busy, but at the end of the day, they work for you as you are coming to them for a service they provide. Later in the book, I will get into how you should be respectful of your prescriber's time to have a detailed conversation about your medication aside from other visits. Just remember, you are the customer. Much like a plumber, the prescriber is providing a service. When you get your taxes done, don't you ask how much they will charge? If you order a steak at a fancy restaurant, do you look to see what the price is before you order? Of course, you do. If you don't, you probably would not be reading this book. Patients MUST become consumers of healthcare, just as they are for other products and services they buy. You see a television on sale in a store and wonder how much it is on Amazon. That is where we need to get with healthcare to drive competition and ultimately get prices down for everyone. The good news is in this book I will show you tools you can use to give you that Amazon like experience in your doctor's office. If your doctor does not seem interested in helping you with this, then it is time to find a new doctor.

Think about the issue from a prescriber perspective for a moment. They read journals, which have ads on every page from manufacturers of new drugs. These many different drugs are peddled as the best things out there, when in most cases, they are only marginally better than the drugs already available. Then they go into their lounge between seeing 30-40 patients, and boom, they see a banner about continuing education sponsored by the newest drug, never a tried and true drug that is effective and economical such as Hydrochlorothiazide, which is the gold standard for high blood pressure treatment.

A recently published survey of prescribers shows that they do not feel that they are responsible for high medication costs. The University of Utah Health survey showed that only 30% of prescribers feel they have a direct impact on costs. This should be alarming to you as a patient! If the prescribers do not feel like they can have an impact on cost, then who will help you? The prescribers surveyed feel that they can't easily determine the price of a drug, and thus they feel powerless on decreasing costs.[12]

Even professional organizations that are supposed to support prescribers, such as the American Medical Association, must show communications from big pharma on novel therapies. Often these new medications are referred to as Me-too drugs. The definition of a Me-too is a drug that is structurally very similar to already known drugs, with only a minor difference. In rare instances Me-too's can create competition and drive down prices, but when this happens, it is often on already inflated brand prices, so even when the prices fall, they are still significantly above the prices of tried and true drugs that are therapeutically equivalent.

Pharmacies also contribute to pricing problems, although to a much lesser extent. As you will find with the tools later in this book, pharmacies do not charge the same price for your medications. The charges can vary greatly from one pharmacy to the next. Important factors include the contract the pharmacy has with the PBM, the usual and customary charge and pharmacies dispensing fees. Large retail chains can in some cases get discounts based on high volumes, but don't forget about your local independent pharmacy for discounts. As I have eluded to there are different generic manufacturers of the same generic drug and depending on where a pharmacy purchases the medication can make a big difference in price. The wholesaler a pharmacy uses can also cause prices to fluctuate. Wholesalers are intermediaries between a pharmacy and a manufacturer who distributes the drugs from point A to point B, while also negotiating pricing in many cases. Finally, pharmacies may have different profit margins based on their niche in the market. An example would be retail pharmacies vs. compounding pharmacies.

Chapter 3 Where Have We Been and Where Are We Headed?

In today's healthcare landscape, prescription drugs make up nearly a quarter of all health insurance premium costs.

According to a report from America's Health Insurance Plans (AHIP).[13], they found that 23.3% of health insurance premium spending goes towards prescription drugs, leaving 76.7% for everything else in the healthcare world, including hospital visits, and you know how expensive those can be. Ten years ago, generic drugs were going to save the day and lower our costs, as many blockbuster brand drugs were ready to go off patent. Well that time has come and gone. The generic wave is over, and we now see some price increases on generic drugs due to reasons laid out in chapter 2. In recent years, the generic drug market has been a race to the bottom. Because of the razor thin margins for generic manufacturers, when the ability to profit dwindles due to new regulations or red tape, the market turns into monopolies and prices start to rise.

A recent example of this was reported by the Wall Street Journal in an article titled "This Form of Zolpidem Tartrate Now Costs Over 800% More." The article outlines how a form of zolpidem (generic of Ambien), a very commonly used sleep aid in nasal spray form[14], increased in price from $69.88 to now $659. The company stated that they were bringing their price in line with other brand name sleep aids, even though they recognized that the nasal spray form was often not covered by insurance and that they were raising prices for a drug that was mostly going to be used by cash paying customers! With generic manufacturers having this line of thinking, it is a good thing you bought this book on how to save your hard-earned money!

"Gag clauses" are another practice you may have heard mentioned in the news of late. This is when pharmacies contract with PBMs to fill scripts in the PBM's network, and in doing so agree to charge the price that the PBM sets for the drug. When a gag clause is in place, the pharmacy must charge the price of the insurance coverage. The gag clause restricts the pharmacy from telling the patient that they could get the drug cheaper by paying cash. They must abide by the contract with the PBM if they are to stay in the network and continue to fill prescriptions for them. Many states have introduced legislation that will ban such clauses, which seem almost criminal. Just days prior to the publishing of this book a federal law was just signed making this practice illegal.

A very important key in this multi-step process is to keep a list of current medications that you can share with any and every healthcare professional you encounter. When you make an appointment to see your doctor, you may see your primary care physician if there is a significant problem that requires their attention, but often you will see a midlevel prescriber, such as a Physician Assistant or Nurse Practitioner. If your Primary Care Physician is unable to see you in a timely manner, you may even go to a clinic site in a grocery store or pharmacy and receive healthcare. If you have a problem that requires a referral, you will likely be referred to a specialist with whom your primary care office is familiar. However, your insurance may want you to see someone in network, or you may read an online review and find another specialist you want to see. Communication between providers can break down during any of these various stages of the process. Too often, a pharmacist will end up seeing multiple prescriptions from multiple doctors or midlevel providers, leading to unnecessary or duplicate prescriptions. If the pharmacist doesn't question this, it can end up costing you big in the end. There is no better way to ensure that care is coordinated between prescribers and other healthcare professionals than to have a list of prescribed medications that each provider can review.

When talking to your doctors about prescriptions, it is also important to advocate your desire to keep medications affordable. You may wonder why prescribers would not give you the most cost-effective prescriptions. Often this comes from not wanting to step on the toes of another prescriber. You must ensure that all providers you see are on the same page for your health and financial wishes, in this order:

1. Safety
2. Efficacy
3. Cost

As you will see in the step-by-step process, you need to take different actions depending on where you are as a consumer of healthcare. A one size fits all model doesn't work for a 45-year-old woman with commercial insurance who has recently been diagnosed with MS and is now going to be taking 3-4 medications versus a 67-year-old man covered by Medicare who takes 15 medications on a maintenance schedule. Wherever you are on the healthcare spectrum, in long term care, home care, soccer mom, or young professional who doesn't take good care of their health, will dictate the steps you need to take. One consistency across all backgrounds is that we all need consumerism in healthcare. We all have a part to play in this. To date we have succumbed to the idea that we have no options. We have one flat copay at the pharmacy, and we must accept whatever drug the doctor(s) have chosen for our issues. Those days are long gone, and we all need to step up and shop for the most economic options that provide similar safety and efficacy. Healthcare currently is a drag on our economy that our employers and government cannot continue to bear. We must introduce a consumerism model to the healthcare system.

As our nation ages, and something in the neighborhood of ten thousand people turn 65 years old every day, more and more adult children end up with the burden of providing home care to elderly parents. If you are in this situation, then you need to look at this book from two angles: one for your own savings potential and one for that of your elderly parents. You might be able to use the savings obtained from the decreased medication costs to hire an aid to help with the care of your aging parents, thus freeing you to continue to work and keep up with the busy life you have beyond the care of the parents.

We have a duty to ourselves, and our nation, to reduce healthcare costs. According to the National Health Expenditure data, the federal government is the largest payer of healthcare, paying more than 28% in 2016.[15] This puts pressure on the federal budget and contributes to rising health insurance premiums. Programs like Medicare and Medicaid are in worse shape than social security at this point, yet nobody seems to be talking about it. As you can see in figure 5, spending on a per capita basis for retail prescription drugs, even adjusting for inflation, has been on a steep increase from 1960 to 2016, according to the Kaiser Family Foundation.[16] This means taxes will have to keep going up or services will have to be reduced to maintain these programs. I encourage you to tell others about this book if you feel it has brought value to you. Spreading the word to friends and family is absolutely worth the effort, as it likely ends up in a win - win situation.

Figure 5

Nominal and inflation-adjusted per capita spending on retail prescription drugs, 1960-2016

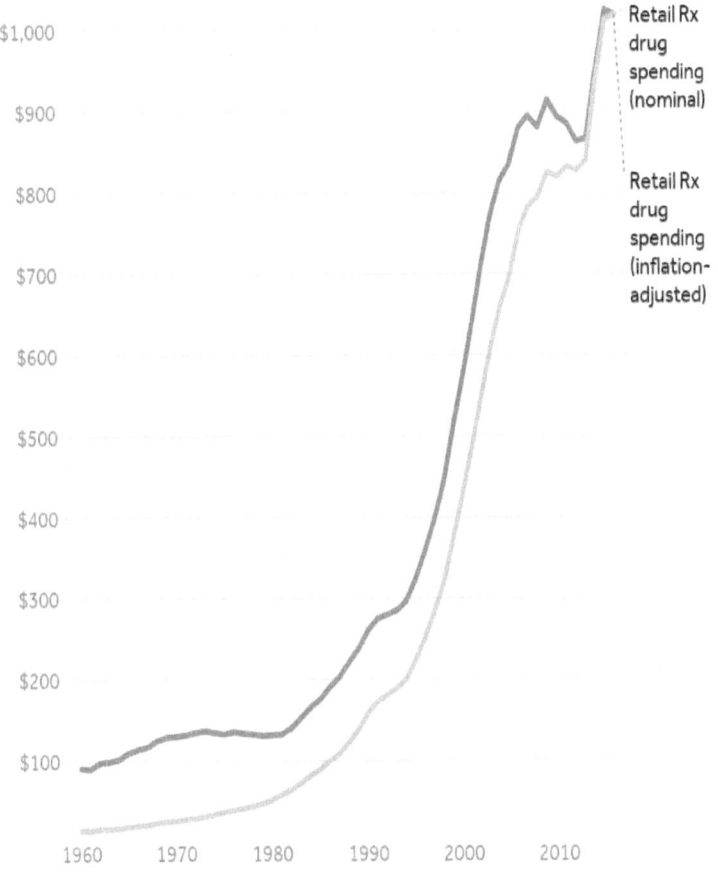

Chapter 4 Insurance Mumbo Jumbo

Have you ever walked up to the pharmacy counter to a disheveled looking pharmacist who has just spent 30 minutes on the phone with your insurance company? They call out your name and communicate to you that there is a problem with your prescription. The drug is non-formulary and thus not covered, but the pharmacist spoke to the insurance; if the doctor completes a prior authorization for step therapy, you may be able to get the drug filled. No guarantees though. Since the drug is in a copay tier 4, and you have hit your deductible limit, your copay for the drug will be a coinsurance percentage. The amount does qualify for reimbursement via your health savings account. The pharmacist then tells you the drug will cost $468 and wants to know if you have your HSA credit card. Are you feeling a bit confused? Join the club.

Health insurance is overly complicated and confusing. You are not alone in the lack of understanding. This kind of scenario was the premise for me writing this book. I realized that most of the health care professionals I worked with had little understanding of how insurance benefits worked and what many common terms meant. If people who work in the healthcare industry are confused, how much more confusing must it be for the average patient. Many people get a crash course once per year in insurance mumbo jumbo when they fill out their open enrollment forms. Health insurance is difficult to understand due to the convoluted way the insurance companies structure the benefits. Too often patients end up just picking a plan because they know their doctor is in it. Because the open enrollment periods last only a couple of weeks, the average person does not feel they have enough time to analyze all the different elements to find which plan might serve them best, and it certainly isn't much fun trying to swim through all the open enrollment paperwork.

Surprising to most, insurance is not always the way to get the best prices on your medications (see the section in Chapter 3 on gag clauses). Our mindset needs to change. We need to think of healthcare insurance like the way most people view homeowner's insurance. You know that if you file a claim on your homeowners' insurance, you may end up getting a higher premium rate, and you will have to pay a deductible. For small fixes on your home, it usually makes more sense to pay for the item on your own, so you will shop around to find the best deal with a good overall value. When purchasing medications, you should look to see what preferred items are on the formulary. If the medication you use is on the formulary, then insurance may be the best route. Otherwise, look to pay cash or use other methods outlined in this book. Whether your medication is on formulary or off, you should be shopping around and looking at the cost of the medication or healthcare service. Taking a little extra time now, could save you and the rest of the population in premiums the next plan year.

Now I will dive into the nuts and bolts of how you can maximize your savings. I have listed many terms in appendix A that you may need help defining and clarifying. I recommend that you flip back to appendix A when you see a word you may not fully understand. Unfortunately, healthcare is full of terminology that is not exactly straightforward. Understanding these keywords will help you when communicating with your doctor and health care team, allowing for optimal results.

Step 1: Medication List

Just as you need a map to find your way to a place you have never been, you will need a map to find your way to prescription savings. Your medication list is your map, and it is critically important to you and your healthcare team. Without the medication list, you have no way to figure out the best route to medication cost savings. Many people reading this book will be on four or more prescription medications, three over the counter products taken regularly, in addition to another three products either prescription, over the counter, or dietary supplements that may be taken on an as needed basis. That is ten products to keep straight, including strength, directions, quantity, pharmacy where you obtain them, who prescribes them and on and on. Do you really expect to keep all that information straight without a list? Now throw in how much those items cost to obtain, remembering all the different price points that may come from shopping at various locations. The list is vitally important and can be made available in a variety of formats. Some of you will want to keep this information in an app on your phone. Others will want a paper backup for your purse or wallet, either typed or handwritten. Still others will want to keep the information in both formats, which is completely fine if you remember to update both versions. I will also address various ways to maintain the list.
Whatever your preference, I have you covered.

The medication list should include all prescription, over the counter, dietary supplements, as well as herbal and homeopathic products that you take daily. You will also need to include any drugs that you take on an as needed basis. Figure 6 below is an example of my customized medication list that contains the key items you need and cuts out what you don't. A full copy is available in appendix B of the book. Additionally, a PDF that can be completed online and printed or saved is available at www.bestrxsavings.com.

Figure 6

www.bestrxforsavings.com **Medication List as of** November 15, 2018

Medication / Strength / Form	Protonix 20mg tablet		
Date Started	May 2018	Color / Shape	Yellow, round
How I take	1 tablet twice a day		
Reason for use	GERD		
Prescriber	Smith	Pharmacy	Hometown Pharmacy

Medication / Strength / Form	Atorvastatin 40mg tablet		
Date Started	2016	Color / Shape	White, oblong
How I take	1 tablet at bedtime		
Reason for use	Cholesterol		
Prescriber	Jones	Pharmacy	Hometown Pharmacy

The medication list requires you to fill out when you started the medication, the medicine dosage, strength and form such as tablet, capsule etc. It has a space for you to note the color and shape. This is to help you identify the pill since many people refer to their meds by description, such as the round white one. This comes in handy, so you can identify the drug when you mix pills in a pill box to help you remember to take them by day. Next, you need to include how you take the medication, one in the morning and two in the evening for example. A very important item on your list is the reason for use. You should know reason for use of every drug! If you do not, please talk to the prescriber, the one who told you to take it (even it if was your neighbor) listed in the next column. Next, be sure to note the pharmacy where you obtain your medication. Finally, the form has a place for you to document any notes and immunizations you have had as those become more prevalent and important in keeping you healthy, especially as you age.

It is important to keep the medication list available for all conversations with your doctor, pharmacist or other healthcare professional. The prescribers' electronic medical records and pharmacies' computer systems will run a Drug Utilization Review (DUR) to ensure your medications have no contraindications, have not been duplicated, and have not been prescribed at too high a dose. Make sure your list matches up with your healthcare teams list so that these computerized programs can help keep you safe and protected from potential drug interactions.

In addition to your medication list, your game changer will be what I call the medication talking points, see a partial example in Figure 7. You can find this form in Appendix C or go to www.bestrxforsavings.com where another workable PDF you can type out online and save, or if you would prefer handwriting the information, simply print it out.

Figure 7

Medication Talking Points
BestRXforSavings.com

Current Medication:

Drug strength & form:	Pristiq		
Started	January, 2018	Who told me to take?	Dr. Smith
Reason for use?	Depression	Helping me?	Not sure
Lifestyle changes	Lose weight	Goal Med to stop	not sure
Side effects?	Weight gain	Can I D/C?	
Current copay	$50	What tier? 3	Other tier cost? $10, $25
365 days /	Days supply 30	= Fills/yr	12
Copay	50	x Fills/yr 12	= Annual Cost $600

Savings options:

Mail Order copay	$25	Mail order days supply	90
365 days /	Days supply 90	= Fills/yr	4
Mail order Copay	$25	X Fills/yr 4	=Annual mail cost $100
Annual cost today	$600	- Annual mail cost $100	=Mail Savings $500

You will complete one medication talking points sheet for every drug on your medication list. Both forms are necessary. The medication list is always with you, while the medication talking points are for your specific conversations with your doctor about meds and cost specifically. I have instructions for every line on the medication talking points form spelled out below in items 1 through 41. I recommend reading through these items briefly now, but don't get hung up. Much more detail is given in the subsequent steps 2-26 of this book about each of the savings methods.

1. Fill in the drug name, strength and form. Example: name= Protonix, strength = 40mg, form = tablets

2. When did you start taking the med? If it has been several years ago, then give an estimate; if the drug is relatively new, put an exact date.

3. Complete who told you to take it: Either the doctor's name or name of person who recommended the medicine if the drug is an OTC or dietary supplement

4. Reason for use: you should be able to complete this from your medication list.

5. Is this helping me? Be honest. In a later step in the process, we will discuss journaling, and if you have had a chance to start that, you can use the information from the journal.

6. Lifestyle changes you can make. (Step 6) Fill in drug you will be able to stop or lower dose of as a result of the lifestyle change.

7. Side effects: Do you have any? Make sure they are due to this drug as much as you can.

8. Can I D/C (discontinue)? Stopping a medication altogether is our first thought for all meds, so we want to have this conversation with the doctor for every medication.

9. What is your current copay for the drug? What price did you pay last time you had this filled at your pharmacy?

10. What is your insurance copay tier? (Step 7)

11. What are the copays for the other tiers per my insurance? (Step 7)

12. Determine a number of fills calculation by completing the numbers on the form.

13. Determine your annual cost by multiplying the copay times the number of fills.

14. Lookup your mail order copay and the days supplied you can get via your insurance; use that to determine the number of fills per year. (Step 13)

15. Determine the annual mail order cost by completing the blanks.

16. Determine the mail order savings.

17. Is the drug generic? (Step 2 to figure out how to tell). If the drug is not generic, is it available as a generic? (Step 11)

18. If the drug is available as a generic, is a $4 generic program available? (Step 11)

19. What is the best cash price? (Step 9) Multiply by the number of fills per year to determine annual cash cost.

20. What is the best OTC price? (Step 7 & 9) Multiply by the number of fills per year to determine annual OTC cost.

21. What is the best discount price? (Step 10) Multiply by the number of fills per year to determine annual cash cost.

22. If drug is not available as a generic (Step 9), then to determine if it is a multi-source brand.

23. List the best multi-source brand price and multiply times number of fills to get best annual price.

24. Larger quantities: use an app or website (Step 14) to lookup larger quantities of your medication and determine pricing. You can also lookup copays for larger supplies via your insurer. Use the best price to do a fills per year calculation and then determine the annual cost.

25. If your med is one that can be split (Step 15), calculate the annual cost using the half tabs.

26. Therapeutic equivalents: (Step 12) use the information to populate the therapeutic equivalent table as described.

27. Do you have an allergy to any of the cost saving therapeutic equivalents? If so, is this truly an allergy or is it something you and your doctor feel you should/could try again while monitoring closely? (Step 18)

28. Combination medication: (Step 16) list out drug / strength / form for each drug. Next, fill in the prices for the combination pills and determine the annual cost. Repeat the step for both insurance copay and cash or discounted prices. Determine annual cost and combination medicine savings based on information from the lines above.

29. Is this medication a combination pill that can be split up? Populate drug/ strength /form and the annual cost from (Step 16) above. Then list out the individual drugs and strengths that can be used to make the combination med. List out the copay and cash prices and determine annual cost by multiplying by number of fills per year. Finally, figure out the annual cost and combination medicine savings per year.

30. Eye drops: determine savings from using eye drops, 1 drop per dose per eye. (Step 17)

31. Nasal sprays: figure savings by using a lower dose with appropriate technique. (Step 17)

32. Oral inhalers: determine savings from a lower dose by using a spacer. (Step 17)

33. Cream/ ointment: determine savings by getting appropriate package size. (Step 17)

34. Samples: (Step 19) and questions to ask your doctor.

35. Patient Assistance Programs: (Step 20)

36. Extra Help Program: (Step 20)

37. State Patient Assistance Program: (Step 21)

38. Medication coupons: (Step 22)

39. Biosimilar: determine if a Biosimilar exists for your medication. (Step 24)

40. Vaccines: list the last administration dates for the vaccines listed. Ask your pharmacist about these prior to meeting with your doctor.

41. Go back and look for the step that yielded the best annual cost from all those that you calculated and highlight it. Focus on this when talking to your prescriber during your medication visit. Show the prescriber that you took the time to do the research on the best option, but don't get bogged down in all the details, as the time in your medication visit will go quickly. Focus on the best route to save for each medication and see the dollar signs dance in your head!

Once you have completed the medication talking points sheets for each drug you take, you will be armed with the expertise to have a conversation with your prescriber about your medications. Knowledge is power, and the knowledge you now have obtained will allow for an effective conversation with your prescriber about your medications. Don't worry not every medication will require you complete all 41 elements, rather this ensures you don't miss anything in the very valuable time you have with your prescriber. This is how you obtain the most cost-effective drug regimen possible.

Step 2: Drug Discontinuation

Never in the history of mankind have there been so many prescription medications available to treat the vast array of diseases and ailments. While advances in medical science are creating great gains in the life expectancy of humans, we are also killing and maiming many via medication adverse side effects. In 2015, the total number of prescription medications filled at pharmacies was just over four billion.[17] That comes out to 13 prescriptions for every person in the United States, per the 2015 census. Additionally, every year the pipeline is full of new drugs coming to the market. The utilization trend is not likely to slow anytime soon unless you start to take a stance that medication is not always the answer.

This high usage comes at a cost. In a study over a 10-year period by the *Journal of the American Medical Association,* results showed that over one third of patients who used medications felt that the medication might have caused depression. The occurrence of depression was higher in patients who took multiple medications. This is significant when you think about the amount of financial and personal stress that an illness already can put on those patients and their families.

The key to Step 2 is to look at your medication list. If you do not know what the medication is being used for, mark it down as a potential medication you can stop. According to consumer reports, 35% of people taking prescription drugs never had a healthcare professional review their medications to see if any could be discontinued.[18] Guess what your savings per year will be if you knock your list down from 10 meds to 6? The savings would be substantial for costs alone but becomes even more substantial when you consider your safety. Do not be afraid to ask your doctor if you can stop a medication. It is likely that if they do not feel you are benefiting, they will say yes. In most cases, they will want feedback from you on if the drug is helping you when they make the decision. According to Consumer Report's 49 percent of survey respondents who regularly take prescription medicine asked their prescribers whether they could stop taking a drug, and 71 percent were able to eliminate at least one. The survey included almost 2,000 adults.

There is an inherent danger in taking some newer branded drugs. Remember as discussed in previous chapters the FDA only looks at safety and efficacy through the first three phases of drug development. Even though that can take several years, they ultimately do not test the drug in a large segment of the overall population. Why is that important? Because when the general population starts taking the drug after the FDA approves it, then patients with all kinds of disease states, backgrounds, genetic makeups that were not part of the FDA review on safety are now able to start this medication. Guess what! You now become a guinea pig to see how the drug works in patients that are not the very tightly controlled groups that the drug company used in their clinical trials. According to the Centers for Disease Control and Prevention, about 1.3 million people went to the emergency room due to adverse effects from medications in 2014. Tragically, 124,000 of those people died!

Have you ever heard of a major FDA recall? In recent years, you have probably seen more and more of these. Recalls show how the FDA neglects to spend enough time in looking at the long-term safety of the medications they approve for the general population. See figure 8 below and ask yourself the following questions: Does the new drug they are talking about in that TV ad that probably costs a tremendous amount of money each month really help my disease state? Could I possibly have a side effect from the drug that the FDA has not yet discovered? Could the drug that I am taking be recalled? If a drug makes it off patent, and the generic becomes available, it means that a much larger safety study occurred. Average people took the medication, and it was at least safe for them, though it may or may not have been effective. The moral of this story is that discontinuing a drug could not only help your wallet but keep you safe as well.

Figure 8[19]

Brand Name	Generic Name	Years on market before withdrawal
Accutane	Isotrentinion	27 years
Baycol	Cerivastatin	3 years
Bextra	Valdecoxib	3.3 years
Cylert	Pemoline	30 years
Darvocet	Propoxyphene / Acetaminophen	55 years
Duract	Bromfenac	1 years
Hismanal	Astemizole	11 years
Lotronex	Alosetron	0.8 years
Meridia	Sibutramine	13 years
Omniflox	Tamafloxacin	0.3 years
Palladone	Hydromorphone E.R.	0.5 years
Posicor	Mibefradil	1 year
Propulsid	Cisapride	7 years
Raptiva	Efalizumab	6 years
Rezulin	Troglitazone	3.2 years
Seldane	Terfenadine	13 years
Vioxx	Rofecoxib	5.3 years
Zelnorm	Tegaserod	4.6 years

Prescription for Maximum Savings

When they FDA reviews a drug for approval, they not only look at safety, but also at efficacy. However, the FDA will not compare the new drug to other existing drugs already on the market that treat the same condition. How do they prove the efficacy of the drug then you ask? Drug companies compare their drug to a placebo (a sugar pill that has no clinical effect at all) to show their drug is more effective than not taking any drug at all. Remember the Me-too's we talked about earlier? These drugs have an effect that is greater than placebo (some much more, others barely more), but may not be anywhere as effective as another drug used to treat the disease. Often these therapeutic equivalents, which have been on the market for longer, are found to be safe and effective for a much lower price. In certain situations, your insurance company will require drugs to go through prior authorization for this very reason. They will try to get you in line with a cheaper, and as effective option. However, to maximize your savings now, you can't wait for your insurance to catch up. You need to try to get these expensive, newer Me too's off your medication list forever. Remember your doctor is not prescribing based on best value. They often do not know the cost of the medication, and they are inundated by advertising from the drug company on the latest and greatest product. The takeaway here is to go through your medication list, find the brand name drugs and mark them, then have a conversation with your doctor about eliminating them. How can you confirm if your drug is brand or generic? Look on your prescription bottle and find the name of the medication. Type this into Drugs@FDA. If the name on your prescription bottle is a generic, you will see a result that shows the same name twice, example: Simvastatin (Simvastatin) your prescription is a brand medication you will see two names. If the name on the bottle matches the first name listed on drugs@fda then you have a brand name medication, example: Zocor (Simvastatin).

The next question to ask is, "Do I still need this drug?" When contemplating if you can discontinue a drug, you need to figure out if it is still working for you. A perfect example of drugs that may no longer be working are the stomach acid blocking drugs known as proton pump inhibitors (PPIs). Millions of Americans rely on PPIs to help with heartburn and gastroesophageal reflux disease better known as GERD. Often due to overeating, overconsumption of alcohol, or a hospital stay, patients will start a PPI. The FDA approved most PPIs for short-term treatment of GERD. Nexium, for example, was approved for one capsule daily for four to eight weeks. These drugs are effective and usually take care of the heartburn; however, when the four to eight weeks is up, they are rarely stopped. In most cases, they are continued on year after expensive year. Do you have a PPI on your profile? Have you ever discussed discontinuing that medication with your doctor at least on a trial basis? You may want to. Not only will it save you the cost of this book many times over, but it may also prevent some long-term side effects related to over suppression of stomach acid, such as lowering bone mineral density, which can lead to Osteoporosis.

I want to make sure you also keep a tally of how much your medications cost you on a yearly basis. Don't get lulled into forgetting that the drug is costing you a ton! Many people are shocked when they look at the annual cost. Is your generic Nexium costing you $30 per month? Well that is $360 per year. Perhaps you are taking a brand name medication such as Viibryd with a monthly copay of $50. You think, "Oh the doctor said I need it, and I can afford $50 per month." Well that totals $600 per year. If you take both medications, you're paying $960 per year for just two medications, and the average American is taking four prescription drugs. That seriously adds up over time. What about a senior on a fixed budget? Does that describe you or your mother or father? Do the positive effects of medications prescribed for dementia or other mental disorders really show enough benefits to justify the large cost? Please take the time to fill in the cost per fill, the number of fills per year, and the annual cost for each of your medications on your Medication Talking Points.

Another problem encountered is that some medications stop working due to progression of the disease state. A drug you were given initially to control your high blood pressure may no longer be effective because you have had a decline in your kidney function. Is it still necessary to be on that medication since your doctor already added a different medication? In other cases, your body will metabolize (breakdown) a drug more effectively after you have been on the treatment for some time. When this happens, instead of upping the dose of the drug as effects begin to decrease due to this higher metabolism, doctors will add another agent. Do you still need to take the first drug? Often the answer is no. Common drugs that fit this profile are alpha-blockers often used for high blood pressure, narcotics that are used for pain, antianxiety medications, and sleep aids. If you can't tell if the drug has an impact on improving the way you feel, then it may be time to have it discontinued.

These are the key questions to ask that will help you figure out what can be discontinued:

1. Do I still have this problem? Journal entries are a key component to answering this question.
2. Am I taking this medication to feed a habit?

Prescription for Maximum Savings

3. Am I having a placebo effect? (Thinking that the drug is helping because I want it to.)
4. Am I experiencing any adverse effects from this mediation?

Step 3: Journaling

How can you be sure if the drug is having a positive effect? For most people it should be easy to tell that I took 600mg of Ibuprofen and now my knee pain is gone. I would say the drug was effective for the problem I was having. However, all too often people don't really remember how they felt before they started the med, and if they have been on therapy a long time, how they felt the first month, or the first year they started using the drug. That is why I strongly encourage you to start journaling about how the medication makes you feel. This does not entail a long-detailed essay on the day's events. Instead, find a time each day that you can jot down anything you noticed, anything that you think could be occurring because of starting a medication, changing the dose of a medication or stopping a medication. This can be as brief as "felt nauseous today before lunch," or "had a headache today right after I woke up." When you look back on these brief notes, then you can start to notice patterns that will help you and your prescriber make sound decisions about if that med is right for you. If it is helping you, it needs to stick around on your med list. If you can't really tell a noticeable difference between before you started taking the med and 30 days later, it might be something to get rid of. Remember some drugs will not actually produce an effect you can sense or feel, for example blood pressure medicine. It is critically important to keep your blood pressure under control to prevent stroke and heart attack, but you will not actually notice a change in how you feel unless your blood pressure was very high before. You need to journal the measure that results from taking the blood pressure medicine. For example, after being diagnosed with high blood pressure, you bought a home blood pressure monitor, and now you take readings once or twice a day. If you journal those readings, it will be very beneficial to your prescriber upon your next visit to see what your reading is on a normal day, and not when you are nervous at the doctor's office getting a reading. With some medication you may only be able to journal if you feel adverse effects, and whether you have to wait for your doctor to draw a lab. Still journaling on those adverse effects will help your overall wellbeing by showing the doctor with actual data why you want to try a different drug, one that is hopefully more economical.

What should you do if you have been taking a medication for a long time but never kept a journal on the medication effects? For the first few weeks, I want you to concentrate on all your medications. Let's say right after you take drug x you feel a little dizzy or maybe it upsets your stomach. Any of these things can provide clues to your prescriber or pharmacist that lets them know you could be having an issue. Maybe the problem is the way you take the medication. A good example would be taking an anxiety med first thing in the morning and then falling asleep at work. All the notes taken over the course of a few weeks could provide valuable insight. Just noting something as a one-time occurrence is less helpful. That is why the journaling is a powerful tool for you to maximize your overall wellbeing. You can go to www.bestrxforsavings.com/resources/ where I have links to a few different journals intended to keep track of your medications. Otherwise, you can use a notebook or notepad; just remember to write the dates in your journal entries.

Step 4: Schedule a Medication Review

At this point, you should feel more confident that you can reduce your drug spending by stopping medications you thought you were doomed to take for the rest of your life. We are still early in the step-by-step process, but at this point, I want you to go ahead and schedule a medication review visit with your doctor. This should be a separately scheduled visit to review your medication talking points only, and not to bring up other issues you are having. The doctor will likely not have any appointments available for at least another week, and that is okay as it will give you time to get through the rest of the steps. Secondly, scheduling the visit now will keep you accountable for getting through the rest of the steps prior to the visit. During the visit, you will start by showing your doctor that you have been researching. Let him or her know that you have done your homework ahead of time; the more knowledgeable you are about your medications, the more likely the prescriber will be to take your concerns to heart. A study from the *Archives of Internal Medicine*, a highly regarded medical journal from 2003, looked at the counseling that doctors gave to patients on medications.[20] The study concluded that the counseling was appropriate only about 18% of the time. That is a shockingly low number, but you must remember that doctors often work in a model where they are paid based on the number of patients they see. This makes it difficult for them to spend extra time during an office visit to discuss medications. Therefore, you need to schedule a visit that is ONLY to talk about medications once you have done your homework, which consists of going through the step-by-step process, preparing your medication talking points, and journaling as discussed above.

One very important final point: once you do your homework, have the visit with your doctor, and identify changes that will help save money, don't be tempted to make too many changes at once. Let your prescriber identify the changes he or she thinks can be made now, those with highest savings first if possible. After a set amount of time confirmed by you and your doctor, look to make another change to help you save. Journaling during this time is critical. You do not want to end up in worse condition for the sake of trying to save some money. Typically, thirty days is a good timeframe to monitor your new medication to ensure there are no ill effects from that change. However, that is dependent on the drug and condition; some could be shorter, some longer.

Step 5: Got Vaccines?

Now that we have talked about how to eliminate as many unneeded medications as possible, I want to review how to eliminate the need for adding any. There have been many articles written on vaccines and their safety. According to the World Health Organization (WHO), immunization through vaccination is the safest way to protect against disease.[21] The WHO goes on to state that it is always best to get vaccinated, even when you think the risk of infection is low. The cost of a vaccination is a fraction of what a hospital stay could end up costing you. In order to maximize savings, you must remember to get vaccinated.

The National Foundation on Infectious Disease states that between 5 to 20 percent of the population can be infected with influenza in any year.[22] Flu vaccination can reduce physician visits, lost work days, and reduce the need for antibiotics. Patients who have Medicare Part B can get influenza, pneumococcal and hepatitis B vaccines at no cost. In fact, more and more insurances are covering these vaccines at no cost, viewing them as preventative. Other important vaccines are Human Papillomavirus or (HPV), which prevents a certain type of cancer, and the shingles vaccine. If you are serious about savings, you need to document when your last vaccination was and follow up with your doctor or pharmacist to see when you are due for a follow up.

The key takeaway here is to ask your prescriber at your Prescription to Save visit, "Do I need any of the following vaccines?"

Prescription for Maximum Savings

1. Influenza - ask every year
2. Pneumococcal - may need more than once
3. Hepatitis B - typically once as an adult
4. HPV - typically once as an adult
5. Shingles vaccine - normally two doses once over 50 years old

Step 6: Lifestyle Changes

You should not always view taking medication as the answer to your problem. Many remedies other than medication could help alleviate the disease state. Diet and exercise may be the two most important things you can do to help lower drug costs since they will allow you to eliminate the need for meds in many cases. Obviously, obesity is an epidemic that must be dealt with; but did you realize that by losing a few pounds, you could reduce the severity of and possibly eliminate diabetes, hypertension, and heartburn, as well as back, knee or hip pain. In many cases exercising and lowering your weight can also help with depression, increase bone mineral density, which prevents osteoporosis, and prevent Dementia or Alzheimer's disease later in life. Simple changes to your diet may also help reduce cases of overactive bladder.

Living a healthier lifestyle can help in other ways too. Excessive alcohol and illicit drug use can cause adverse effects when mixed with many prescriptions and over the counter medications. According to *Medical News Today*, the top 10 causes of death in the United States are the following:[23]

1. Heart disease
2. Cancer
3. Chronic lower respiratory disease
4. Accidents
5. Stroke
6. Alzheimer's disease
7. Diabetes
8. Influenza and pneumonia
9. Kidney disease

10. Suicide

Nine out of the ten items on this list have modifiable factors; a lifestyle change can often help to prevent death from these causes. Long-term chronic care for patients who suffer from these diseases can cost trillions of dollars. To help prevent these costs, your health insurance will pay for certain screenings, prenatal care, coaches or personal nursing, or pharmacy care, along with discounted services such as gym memberships. My advice here, investigate these benefits and use them.

The Centers for Disease Control and Prevention estimates more than 36% of U.S. Adults have obesity.[24] This is expected to balloon to 50% by 2030 if something is not done to stop the trend. Sixty other chronic conditions are linked to obesity, and it is estimated that obesity accounts for 20% of annual health care costs. Campaign to End Obesity is a great resource to find a wealth of information on this topic, and I encourage you to look at the valuable information on this site if you are struggling with obesity. Dieting is hard and having a support system around you to help you and hold you accountable for meeting goals is one of the best things you can do to meet your goals. Weight loss goals should include the following; I want to lose x number of pounds by x date, and I want to be able to eliminate my high blood pressure medication or one of my medications to lower my blood sugar. A recent article by CNBC highlights diets that have defeated Diabetes. I would encourage you to read up on how new fresh-food prescriptions are beating pricey drugs.[25]

The next lifestyle modification may be the single most important piece of advice I, can give you. If you are a smoker, and you want to spend less on your medications, you must stop smoking. I know it is an addiction, and I would never advocate for quitting without appropriate resources, such as some form of nicotine replacement therapy and a large support structure, including family, friends, and accountability partners. Smoking accounts for 80% of COPD related deaths.[26] When you look at the math, quitting smoking itself would be a huge financial windfall. The average smoker smokes one pack per day. At the time of this writing, a pack of cigarettes cost about $7 per pack with taxes. That means it costs $49 per week to smoke, which comes out to $2548 per year! If your boss said you were getting a $2500 raise, wouldn't you take it? That doesn't even include the savings on your health insurance, as some companies are now asking employees who smoke to pay more for their coverage. In addition, the price of life insurance increases if you are a smoker. Other added costs include expensive inhalers for those who acquired COPD, not to mention frequent bouts of pneumonia and other lung infections that run up costs from trips to urgent care or, worse, the emergency room, along with antibiotic costs to treat the infection itself. Continue to smoke long enough, and it can cause sleep issues for you and your spouse; you might even end up with a CPAP machine to help you breathe, which is very expensive. In addition to the monetary savings, quitting smoking will prevent more heart attacks and strokes than any cholesterol medication. It will also allow you to avoid emphysema, chronic bronchitis, cancer of the lung, mouth, esophagus, bladder and larynx for you and family members, as second-hand smoke can harm those around you while you smoke. If you want to save money, the choice is clear; you need to stop smoking.

The positive effects of exercise or any physical activity can't be stressed enough. You don't have to run a marathon. Taking a walk, gardening or anything that gets you up and moving and gets your heart rate up is going to pay dividends when it comes to your overall health. You don't have to wait until the beginning of the year, month or week. Getting any activity going is the key. Do something that you can build on over time. The importance of a routine can't be overemphasized. It doesn't matter if it is in the morning, at lunch, or in the evening... Just start it. It would be much easier to walk using a device that tracks steps than to have to take an expensive medication. The gold standard in medicine for evaluating someone's risk of heart attack or stroke comes from the Framingham Risk Model. The Framingham Risk Score was first developed based on data obtained from the Framingham Heart Study, which estimated a person's 10-year risk of developing coronary heart disease.[27] The Heart Study found that the most physically active patients, which consisted of the top ⅓ of study participants, had a 40% lower death rate than the lower ⅔. Being in poor physical shape is a very dangerous thing!

Most people do not take sleep seriously enough. Insomnia caused by poor sleep hygiene has been linked to many adverse health effects. Sleep hygiene is a variety of different practices and habits that are necessary to have a good night's sleep and full daytime alertness. It consists of important steps like having your room dark, quiet, and set at a good temperature. It includes not lying in bed for long periods before going to sleep, turning the television off, and keeping ambient light such as from your cell phone out of your face before bed. Going to bed at about the same time every night and trying to get 7.5-8 hours of sleep per night all make for good sleep hygiene. Also, you should not eat hot spicy food and not drinking caffeine 3-4 hours before going to bed will also help you be able to get and stay asleep.

Sleep is a key ingredient to overall health. Research has proven that not enough sleep or interrupted sleep can increase the risk for diseases such as high blood pressure, obesity, diabetes and heart disease.[28] Additionally, numerous studies have shown that sleep deprived people often test out in a similar way to someone who would be considered legally intoxicated. Drowsiness due to poor sleep has attributed to thousands of crashes per year. Want to run up your medical expenses, try getting in a car accident!

Obviously, the best path is to make a concerted effort to get good quality sleep; it will pay dividends in the long run.

On the lifestyle section of your Medication Talking Points, you should document what lifestyle changes you will attempt to make. Think carefully about your goals prior to your visit with your doctor to review your medications. During the appointment let your doctor know what changes you are planning to make to your lifestyle and discuss what if any medications you might be able to eliminate if you can stay on track. Your doctor might be able to suggest counseling or other support services to assist you in your effort to achieve those goals.

Step 7: How Do I Save Using my Insurance?

Now that you have created your medication list, identified medications that might be candidates for discontinuation, and thought about lifestyle changes that you can use to eliminate even more medication, you are ready for the next step. You need to calculate the annual cost for your medication. Something drew you into reading this book, and it was likely that you knew that you had been spending too much on medication. But do you know exactly how much? Determining your annual medication costs will allow you to give your doctor a verified reason why you made the appointment to talk specifically about your medications. It will also help you to determine where the areas of opportunity lie. To calculate your annual medication cost per year, follow the formula below.

On your medication talking points, you will see a column that denotes how often you are getting the medication refilled. First note the number of days supplied by the medication; some common examples are 30, 60, and 90 days. Next figure out the number of fills you will need for the year. For example, if the prescription is for 30 days and you take the medication every day then you would get the medication filled once every month, and you would mark 12 in this column. The final step is to document how much you paid for the script at the quantity you last purchased, which was your day's supply. Now multiply the amount paid x the number of fills per year to get your annual cost.

Example: $25 x 12 fills per year = $300 annual cost

Once you figure up your annual costs, you can figure out which medications you need to reconsider to lower your annual cost. First things first, figure out if you are maximizing your savings using your insurance. To do this you have to look at the formulary to determine the copay tier of the drugs you take. In some cases, your medication may be excluded, and the formulary will tell you that. You will have copay tiers that typically look like this example:

Generic $5
Formulary preferred brand $25
Formulary non-preferred brand $50
Non-formulary $150

As you can see, where the drug falls in the formulary of your insurance carrier can have an extreme difference in your out of pocket costs. How can you figure out where the drug falls per your insurance? Probably the easiest place to look is at the enrollment material, which will give you a breakdown of these formulary tiers. If you don't have that information anymore, well never fear, it's the internet to the rescue. You can look on the site of your insurer and try to figure this out. Sometimes you will need to check the website of the pharmacy benefit manager (PBM) that your insurer uses. You should have received a letter in the mail after you enrolled that told you what website to look at for medication information. Most websites will already have your drugs you have had filled in some type of display that should tell you what the tier is. That site may also list some cost saving measures you can take to be more in line with the formulary. What if you have never been on the website before or you have lost the letter? The next option if you are web savvy is to google your insurance. You should look at your prescription membership card and google the name on the card then add the word "formulary" to the search. You should find a list pop up for your insurer that gives a list of commonly prescribed drugs and where they stand on the formulary. If you don't like to use the internet, you can use the alternate route of calling to speak to your benefit provider. You will want to call the number on the back of your prescription drug card, the same one you would give to the pharmacy when you go to get a script. Before you make this call, you will want to have your medication talking points filled out as completely as you can, so you can get through all your questions when you talk to a representative. Regardless of whether you do this online or by calling, you will want to find out what drugs are the preferred brands or generics they are recommending and document this to aid in the conversation with your prescriber during your visit to discuss savings.

In many cases, certain drugs will be not covered by your insurance. What does that mean to you exactly? It means you are responsible for the full cost of the medication. Often this will happen when they are trying to prescribe you something that is available as an over the counter medication (OTC). Many insurers will try to deflect the cost of those medicines to the patient. Some drugs are available in both OTC and prescription strengths; for example, ibuprofen 200mg is OTC, but Ibuprofen 400mg, 600mg and 800mg are all prescription. Some insurances will say that a prescription written by your doctor for ibuprofen 800mg is not covered because they want you to buy the over the counter version, which you would need to take 4 x 200mg tablets to get your 800mg dose. You need to keep track of this spending on the OTC drugs, as they can be counted toward your deductible, which I will discuss later in the book.

When you go in to look for OTC drugs in the pharmacy, it is important to keep in mind that you do not want to get brand name products if possible. Check store brands because they will usually be a better deal than other manufacturers of OTC drugs, much as grocery store brands are often cheaper than name brands on grocery items. If the doctor wrote you a prescription for Robitussin for example, you want to look at what the active ingredient is in Robitussin, which is Guaifenesin for plain Robitussin. If you look just to the right or left of Robitussin on the shelf, you will find a generic Guaifenesin product at a much lower price. Remember OTC drugs must undergo safety and efficacy testing by the FDA, so you can feel confident with store brands.

There can be other reasons why a drug is not covered by insurance. This can happen to prescription medications as well, not just OT C drugs. When you find out that a drug is not covered, and it is only available as a prescription, you will want to investigate what the other options are on the formulary. Otherwise, you will be responsible for the full cost of the medication. Why do insurers set up the benefit in this way? Well there are many reasons, but they get better deals when formulary agents are used, so it helps them keep your premiums lower. The shock of being told the full price of the drug at the pharmacy often leads to something termed prescription abandonment. This is where the patient leaves without getting the prescription filled. Many times, the prescriber is unaware of this until their next interaction with the patient, and that can lead to negative outcomes for the disease state in many cases. According to an article written in the *Annals of Internal Medicine*, 36% of prescriptions that are rejected by the payer end up being abandoned.[29] By doing your homework and being knowledgeable of the drugs that are on your formulary, you can prevent having to abandon your prescriptions.

Your prescriber may feel that a drug that is not on formulary or that has prior authorization requirements is necessary. These requirements are put in place to ensure that the drug is being used for the correct reasons and for the right disease state. The insurer may also want you to use a different product in the same drug class. If the result of the prior authorization is that the request was denied, you or your doctor can appeal the decision. If you or your doctor can provide information to the insurer that the drug is medically necessary, the insurer will do an independent medical review of the appeal. That appeal could lead to your drug being covered after all. The processes I have described above should keep you from running into these situations, but sometimes it can't be avoided. The key to remember is to NOT just pay out the nose for a drug that was denied in the prior authorization process. File the appeal or ask your doctor to on your behalf. Every insurer has an appeal process, and if they don't provide you information on how to do the appeal, then you can look at the state appeal rights. To file a state appeal, google search prior authorization appeal rights in the state where you live and fill in the blanks. If you find yourself in this situation, you will want to make sure to check out later steps in the process.

Step 8: Are You a Veteran?

According to the US Census Bureau there are 19 million veterans in the United States.[30] Those brave men and women have some advantages when it comes to paying for prescription medications. The VA model for drug coverage for veterans is one area where the government has done a good job in providing benefits. Unlike Medicare and Medicaid, the VA contracts with pharmaceutical companies to use their size to drive medication pricing. The VA can negotiate lower prices and larger discounts for drugs across most therapeutic classes. Additionally, they have a robust formulary that helps members have access to important therapies at relatively good prices.

The VA assigns members to different priority levels according to various differing factors. These can include income, medical conditions, and if the conditions were tied to military service. Military treatment facilities offer most medications at low or no cost. Veterans also have the option of getting prescriptions through TRICARE mail order pharmacy. If you had an honorable discharge, you can get mail order scripts for low or no charge. You can confirm your eligibility on the TRICARE website at www.tricare.osd.mil/. One problem for patients who are enrolled at lower priority levels is they could be in jeopardy of losing some benefits if federal funding declines. In 2017, a tiered copay medication structure (TCMS) went into place. It established copays for 30-day prescriptions of $5, $8 and $11 for Tiers 1-3 respectively. This includes some OTC drugs as well. Veterans who are in priority groups 2 through 8 have a $700 annual copay maximum. The program could be very valuable for you, and you can use the website https://www.pbm.va.gov/ to check prices online.

Some patients are confused when it comes to Medicare and VA benefits. They are separate, and you should always use your VA benefits at a VA facility. Even if you are Medicare eligible, you are still eligible for TRICARE. This is important because your VA drug coverage is better and less costly than Medicare. You should still consider signing up with a Medicare Part D drug plan in case you need to get medical care outside of a VA facility. This could be very important. If you are not near a VA facility and must get treatment at a non-VA facility, you could be on the hook for the entire bill! Having both types of medical coverage gives you more options for finding the best deals on medication and allows for covered treatment outside of VA facilities.

Finally, the VA has many financial assistance options. They have waiver options and various types of payment plans. You can also apply for a hardship determination to get exemptions on copayments, sometimes up to a year. This can be especially helpful in cases where income changes drastically from one year to the next, as could happen if you were unable to work because of a disease. You can find more information at https://www.va.gov/healthbenefits/resources/publications/hbco/hbco_copayments.asp

Step 9: Could it be Cheaper to Pay Cash?

Should you always use your insurance benefits? Many people think that because you have insurance, you must use it. Do you remember when I said before that we should try to get into the mindset of using health insurance like homeowner's insurance, only when you really need it? Well, in many cases you will find that not using your health insurance and just paying cash, also known as self-pay, might be a better deal for you. In fact, in a letter from the *Journal of the American Medical Association* in March 2018, researchers looked at 9.5 million prescription claims from Medicare Part D and found that a patient's copayment was higher than the cash price for 1 in 4 drugs.[31] Additionally, for 12 of the 20 most commonly prescribed drugs, those overpayments were higher by more than 33%. See an illustration of this in figure 9. The amount of overpay is the reason that some pharmacy benefit managers institute gag clauses on pharmacies as they are collecting the copay amount, and what is done with the additional monies is not disclosed.

Figure 9

Cost of Drug	*$11.65*
Pharmacy dispensing fee	*$2.00*
Tax	*$0.95*
Total	*$14.60*
Copay amount	*$50.00*
Amount overpaid	**$35.40**

A recent study done by *Consumer Report*'s secret shoppers found that a 30 day supply of a common medication varied greatly in price based on location.[32] For 25 different independent pharmacies and the major national chain pharmacies, the cost range was $69-$1351. That shows how important this step can be in the process. You must be vigilant about checking on prices of your medications in order to maximize your savings.

Step 10: Drug Discount Programs

How can you find out for sure what the cash price is? Well in today's technological age, you have a multitude of websites and apps at your disposal. The first to check out is GoodRx. They have a website and mobile app that is easy to use and offers coupons, shows prices at various retail stores in your area, and maps them out for you. GoodRx claims to save consumers up to 80% on prescriptions. Typically, if you buy your script with cash, the pharmacy does not submit a claim to your insurance. Therefore, your insurance does not know that you are getting that medication filled. The discounted prices are what the PBM has negotiated with the pharmacy in question, and GoodRx is giving you visibility into that. Additionally, they provide coupons that are not manufacturer coupons but GoodRx discount coupons. Manufacturer coupons will be discussed later in the book. The pharmacy runs these claims through the GoodRx service to track and, in some cases, report back to the manufacturers, who also may pay them for the service.

Another good tool is Blink Health. The Blink model is a little different. They negotiate directly with manufacturers to get a lower price. As of this writing, they only have around 15 thousand drugs in scope for discounts, so not all drugs are included. Some generics and some high-priced brands haven't contracted with Blink Health, so they will not have savings opportunities.

The third mobile app I will bring up is WeRx, which is a price comparison tool that allows you to see the differences in prices at local pharmacies for your prescribed medications. You can see on your smartphone a map of different prices in different areas around you. It also allows you to share and compare local and online prices

These third-party drug discount sites such as GoodRx.com, BlinkHealth.com and WeRx negotiate discounts on drugs with pharmacy benefit managers who adjudicate claims. That means when you present your discount card for your prescription, the pharmacy will find out from the PBM the negotiated price and charge that price to you. They may claim these are coupons, but they are just drug discount programs. You may wonder why pharmacies participate in these discount plans. Pharmacies hope to bring you and others into their pharmacy through these discount programs and, while you are in the store, sell other items to you as well. Therefore, it is worth your time and effort to investigate prices using these apps.

Drug discount programs are available from a variety of sources, not just mobile apps. These discount cards should be free and are downloadable, so they can be presented at any pharmacy that accepts the discount card. When your pharmacist fills your prescription, they will use the adjudication information on the card to process the claim and give you the discounted price, just like with the mobile applications. These discount cards can save you money on brand and generic drugs. The best place to find out about these is through online searches. There are no restrictions on obtaining discount cards and that makes them easier to obtain than manufacturer coupons or patient assistance programs (PAP) programs that will be discussed later. These discount programs can reduce your out of pocket costs for drugs not covered by your insurance or with other insurance restrictions such as prior authorization or quantity limits. Some discount programs offer better deals than other discount programs, so it is worth your time to search for more than one. Keep in mind that the prices are subject to change and can do so frequently. The prices you see in apps or online are estimates, and due to a variety of factors, will not be the exact price you will pay, though it should be close. Finally, keep in mind that your doctor and pharmacist are not likely to know much about these discount programs. They may know they exist but not a whole lot more than that.

Numerous drug discount programs exist, and I am not going to try to give you an exhaustive list. The apps described above are the easiest to use if you have a mobile phone and like that type of convenience. To make the steps in this process as easy as possible, it is necessary to introduce you to a site that will have multiple uses across several steps. That site is NeedyMeds.org. When you visit the site, you go under the patient savings tab, and then additional resources to lower costs and you will see the Needymeds drug discount card. Their drug discount card claims to save you up to 80% on cash prices of not only prescription but also over the counter medications. You need to ask your doctor for a prescription even if the drug is an over the counter medication. This will assist you in being able to use the discounts for these drugs. These discounts can be used by anyone but can't be combined with insurance. You can use this in place of your insurance and pay cash for the remaining cost after the discount. NeedyMeds tracks how many times you use the card and the amount of savings realized, but it is anonymous. This means they do not track your information with those savings amounts. You can search for pharmacies that accept the NeedyMeds discount on the website and check drug pricing. They also offer an app called storyline that has many features, but most importantly allows you to check prices and has the discount card built in for you to use at the pharmacy. Prescriptions for pets are also available for these discounts, and they have information on the website about how to use this feature.

Checking medication prices on all these apps is simple and takes very little time. Your medication talking points should be available with the names of the medications you need to get prices on. It really doesn't hurt to run prices via these sites for all your medications to see if any surprise deals pop up. Once you find the best deals, make sure to note them on your medication talking points along with the pharmacy offering that price. You will need to try to negotiate price matches at the pharmacy that you prefer, but that will come later after you have completed a few more steps.

Figure 10 describes some other good drug discount resources. This is by no means a full list of apps and or websites as more are appearing all the time.

Figure 10

FamilyWize Community Service Partnership	*Works with nearly all pharmacies nationwide and negotiates prescription discounts with them. Their discount cards have no restrictions and can lower medication costs by up to 75%.*
RxSavingsPlus	*Prescription discount program for non-insured or non-covered drugs. Accepted at thousands of pharmacies nationwide. They provide you with a discount card with savings of up to 70% with the average savings of 22% off regular retail prices. This can be used anytime a drug is not covered by insurance and can be used for your entire family, including pets.*

Step 11: Generics

The next step in the process is to look for generic drugs when possible. In step one, you should have written down your medication list and looked at if the medications you were taking were name brand or generic. For all those on the list that were name brand, you need to walk through this step. If you had only generics listed, you can skip to the next step. Typical insurance benefits charge lower copays for generic drugs. They are less expensive for you and your insurer. You may have copay tiers in your prescription benefits, and generics are typically the lowest tier, which is going to be the lowest cost copay to you. They are trying to encourage you to use their lowest cost option by making them your lowest copay tier.

There are over ten thousand generic drugs listed in the FDA's Orange book. The Orange book contains drug products with therapeutic equivalence that the FDA has approved based on safety and effectiveness. If a generic drug is not listed in this book, your pharmacist cannot interchange it with the brand name drug. I discussed generics in previous chapters; the key takeaway is to know that many retail and mail order pharmacies offer $4 generic programs. The name has evolved over time, and some pharmacies will now offer free generics, some $4 for 30-day supply, and some $15 for 90-day supply. Various programs exist, and some require enrolling as a member or paying an annual membership, so you need to read the fine print. With so many programs available, I would encourage you NOT to pay an annual fee. Check around to various pharmacies, and don't forget the independent pharmacies, often smaller pharmacies will offer these programs or price match to keep your business. You need to communicate your dosage as well to ensure that it is covered; occasionally high dosages will not be available for the discounted $4 generic programs. Continually ask your doctor and pharmacist if there is a generic available for the drug(s) on your medication list. You should also ask your pharmacy if they have added any new generics to the $4 discount programs.

Once a drug becomes generic, there will only be one generic manufacturer for the first 6 months. Then after that, more generic manufacturers can come into the mix, increasing competition and driving prices down further.

One more thing to note when searching for generics that can render your savings is that some products that are brand name are referred to as multisource. Multisource means that more than one pharmaceutical manufacturer selling a drug containing the same active ingredient in the same dosage form. One example of this is the chemical, diltiazem, originally introduced to the market as the brand name product Cardizem. Generics exist for the Cardizem version of diltiazem. Then other brand products were introduced to the market, which were long acting, so the drug could be dosed once or twice per day versus four times a day like the original Cardizem product. These exist under the brand names Cartia XT, Cardizem CD, Tiazac, Diltia XT, Taztia and Dilacor XR. Each of these brands has one or many generics. However, the generic for Cardizem CD can't be interchanged for Diltia XT. Some other commonly prescribed multisource drugs are listed here in Figure 11.

Figure 11

Cardizem	Clozaril	Coumadin	Dilantin	Diltiazem	Dilt XR
Gengraf	Glucophage XR	Glumetza	Lanoxin	Levoxyl	Neoral
Sandimmune	Synthroid	Tiazac	Tegretol	Unithroid	Zarontin

Multisource drugs can get complicated, so be sure to talk to your pharmacist if you have questions on the specific generic for the form of a multisource drug you are taking. Remember this can save you a LOT of money, so don't forget to have this conversation with your doctor. Doing your research and knowing this information ahead of your conversation with your doctor will show him or her that you are serious about controlling medication costs and will make these decisions easier for your doctor to make. Your doctor will appreciate that. Having your doctor's appreciation will help with the next item on the list, having a conversation about any brand name medications you take that might be tagged as dispense as written (DAW) by your prescriber. Dispense as written (DAW) means the brand is medically necessary. It is a communication from your doctor to the pharmacist that generic substitution is not allowed. This can be a costly thing for your doctor to do, and if there are drugs that they have marked as DAW, you will need to have a conversation with your doctor to understand the reason behind the decision. One common example of this is narrow therapeutic index drugs may cause your prescriber to want to stay with a branded product. These are drugs that have a small range between being effective and having dangerous side effects, figure 12 lists some examples of narrow therapeutic index drugs. Often it is true that changing back and forth from brand to generic can have adverse effects on your treatment and is not a good option. However, don't be fooled into thinking you have to be on the brand forever. Typically, prescribers are looking for consistency with these medications. They want you on the brand or on a generic consistently. Be ready to commit to your prescriber that you will not be moving back and forth from brand to generic, or to generics from different manufacturers. Something you may have to work with your pharmacist to ensure consistency. Also, plan to be closely monitored for any issues that arise when moving from brand to generic. This may cost you an extra office copay or two, but in the long run, you could save big on your medications. A good example of this is when taking certain medications for organ transplantation. These will need to be closely monitored, and the key is to buy only small amounts to start, even of the generic you are trying to switch to, so you can confirm it works for you and doesn't cause adverse effects.

Figure 12

Generic Name	Brand Name
Carbamazepine	Tegretol
Cyclosporine	Neoral or Sandimmune
Digoxin	Lanoxin
Ethosuximide	Zarontin
Levothyroxine	Synthroid
Lithium	Eskalith
Phenytoin	Dilantin
Procainamide	Procanbid
Theophylline	Theodur
Warfarin	Coumadin
Tacrolimus	Prograf

Step 12: Therapeutic Equivalents

This step is one of the most important tools in your toolbox to reduce costs. To put it simply not all medications are available as a generic. When that is the case, you need to look at drugs that are therapeutic equivalents, meaning they have essentially the same effect in the treatment of a disease as one or more other drugs. While it is not chemically equivalent, the effect should be similar. These drugs work by a similar mechanism of action; an example would be drugs classified as diuretics. They all will make you produce more urine via your kidneys to help lower your blood pressure, but some work on different parts of your kidney to create this effect.

Many times, in this book, I have referenced drugs dubbed as Me-too's. Drugs that come out with similar mechanism of action as products that are already on the market but are often much more expensive. A classic example of this is the drug Duexis. Originally marketed for treatment of pain due to rheumatoid arthritis or osteoarthritis, it contains two commonly prescribed drugs, famotidine and ibuprofen. Famotidine (Pepcid) suppresses stomach acid and ibuprofen (Motrin) is a commonly used anti-inflammatory. When you consider that 90 tablets of Duexis, which lasts for one month, costs $2400 or more while you can get the two separate component drugs in any pharmacy for less than $20, you must wonder why Duexis would ever be warranted.

Blood pressure lowering drugs are a prime example of medications with many therapeutic equivalents available. The governing body that sets treatment guidelines for hypertension (high blood pressure) is known as the Joint National Committee (JNC) on Prevention, Detection, Evaluation and Treatment of High Blood Pressure. They regularly update their guidelines with the most up to date medical information from clinical trials with thousands of patients. The most recent release is called JNC 8 guidelines.

Their updates discuss treatments that are first line agent's vs those that are second line or reserved for patients with other special circumstances. The idea is to have a guideline for treatment of a disease that affects millions of people as hypertension does and offer a tool prescribers can use to try to treat the disease in the most effective manner as proven by mountains of literature and study. Those JNC guidelines point to first line therapy as thiazide diuretics for the initial treatment of the disease.[33] What do these wonder drugs cost? The most common drug in that class is a generic called hydrochlorothiazide and it costs... drumroll... $4 for a 30-day supply in most pharmacies. Compare that to many other options used to treat high blood pressure and you will find a wide variance from that price. I am not trying to imply that every patient will be able to manage hypertension with hydrochlorothiazide alone, but your doctor should have at least started from that point based on the JNC 8 guidelines. Don't worry if hydrochlorothiazide doesn't work for you though, the other three classes stated by JNC 8 as initial drugs of choice are ACE inhibitors, Angiotensin receptor blockers and calcium channel blockers. Each of those classes of drugs has a very cheap generic option available. So, if you are spending a lot of money on the newest drug out there for high blood pressure, please ask your doctor about a therapeutic equivalent in one of these classes of drugs. Your prescriber may be reluctant to change your medicine if it seems to be working, following the "if it isn't broke don't fix it" mentality. However, if you can no longer afford the medication then something needs to be done, regardless of how good the blood pressure readings are. Don't be afraid to have the conversation with your doctor about therapeutic equivalents. They will be on your side if you tell them about your real need to avoid overspending.

Hypertension is not the only disease state that can offer savings by using therapeutic equivalents. In fact, almost all disease states can. The Medical letter on drugs and therapeutics said that depression medications known as SSRIs have no difference in efficacy.[34] The real rationale for selecting one of the drugs in that class comes down to adverse effects, drug interactions and cost. See the chart in figure 13 depicting how generic therapeutic equivalents can save you a tremendous amount of money.

Figure 13

Drug	Quantity per 30 day supply	Cost
Citalopram (Celexa) 20mg	30	$7.08
Escitalopram (Lexapro) 10mg	30	$10.75
Fluoxetine (Prozac) 20mg	30	$5.30
Paroxetine (Paxil) 20mg	30	$7.00
Sertraline (Zoloft) 50mg	30	$10.89
Vilazodone (Viibryd) 20mg	30	$262.68

Several novel new therapies have been found for treating blood clots. However, these drugs come with very large price tags as you can see in figure 14, especially when compared to generic warfarin.

Figure 14

Drug	Quantity for 30 day supply	Cost
Pradaxa 150mg	60	$387.14
Xarelto 20mg	30	$424.69
Eliquis 5mg	60	$424.65
Savaysa 30mg	30	$342.79
Bevyxxa 80mg	30	$467.75
Warfarin (Coumadin) 5mg	30	$7.43

You prescriber might be lured into prescribing one of these medications for you in hopes that the cost of your overall healthcare spending will go down. How is that you ask? The therapeutic alternative here is warfarin, which is a generic. It is a tried and true effective treatment for conditions such as atrial fibrillation, deep vein thrombosis (DVT), pulmonary embolism (PE) and other blood clotting disorders. What is the concern? Well warfarin requires that you stay within a certain lab value range termed the international normalized ratio or INR, which is a measure of how long it takes your blood to clot. If you are too low, you are still at risk for a blood clot; if too high, you risk for bleeding problems, the worst of which could be a stroke. However, if you are monitored and stay within the range, warfarin is quite successful in preventing blood clots. You would need to talk to your doctor and determine if it would save you money to be closely monitored or to be on the more expensive drug where monitoring is not required. The monitoring consists of getting blood drawn and talking with your prescriber or pharmacist about your diet, adherence to taking the medicine, and other drugs you are taking. Many times, if you find a warfarin clinic that is typically managed by pharmacists you can be very well managed and save money by not having to pay for the expensive drug. Again, the tradeoff is the monitoring, which can be anywhere from three to four times a week in the beginning and while adjusting the dose to every two to three weeks once your level is stabilized.

Another target for therapeutic equivalents is in diseases states or conditions where the outcome is not measured by a lab value. This is often referred to as a subjective outcome as it is up to the patient to describe how they feel. This goes back to the importance of journaling on your medications. The only true way to remember accurately how the drug is affecting you is by writing it down daily or when some effect, good or bad, is noticed by you. Then once you go back and look at what you have noted about the medication over time, you can decide if you need a change. If you notice it has no effect, or you don't really notice symptoms of the condition or disease, then you can eliminate the drug as was mentioned in Step 2. However, if you are still having problems due to the disease state, then it is time to look for a therapeutic equivalent. Typically, you should be able to find one that is more cost effective as well, and that fact alone may have a positive placebo effect on you, just knowing you are benefiting financially.

Certain disease states require discretion on selecting therapeutic alternatives. Some examples include cancer, seizures, heart arrhythmias, HIV, and Hepatitis C. The management of these disease states often require specialist physicians. They are the experts in the field, but never be afraid to ask for lower cost options. Given the fact that you will often not have as close of a relationship with a specialist as you will with your primary care doctor, you need to insist this doctor work with you to keep medication spending down. Often these disease states have drugs that are very expensive and can be the most impactful way for you to realize cost savings.

When you have identified on your medication talking points that the drug is a brand with no generics available, mark that down as a candidate to look for therapeutic alternatives. To determine if therapeutic alternatives are available, you can simply google the drug name and then therapeutic alternatives. You should see several reference pages such as drugs.com or others that will list therapeutic alternatives if they exist. Write down the names and then call or stop by to see your pharmacist. Tell them you are looking for therapeutic alternatives for your medications and want to know if the list you found online would be good options. The ones that your pharmacist says would be viable options are the ones you will want to talk with your doctor about at your medication appointment. Don't take the entire list you find online into the appointment with the doctor and expect to get through everything in the allotted time. Your pharmacist is a valuable free resource when searching for these alternatives, and you should use their expertise.

Step 13: Pharmacy Types

Not all pharmacies are the same in terms of price. The chain pharmacies that you have seen buying up small independent pharmacies and building a new store on seemingly every corner are not always the best place to get a deal on your medications. For the purpose of simplicity, I am going to break out pharmacy types in the following way: retail chains, specialty pharmacies, mail order pharmacies, independent pharmacies, which may be one store or have several locations in a region, and online pharmacies.

Retail chains can be comprised of national retailers, drug story only stores, grocers and large box stores. While these pharmacies certainly have purchasing power based on size, that doesn't always mean you will find the best deal at these pharmacies. Many of these pharmacies are a way to drive the customer into the store where they hope you will then buy other items in the store, which creates higher profit margins. This is likely the reason that in general Costco is one of the best values in this pharmacy type. You can always google drug prices at Costco or look on the wall in the store where signs will often have the names of commonly used drugs that they have at often deeply discounted prices. You do not need a membership to enter the store and use the pharmacy, although they may have further benefits for you if you do. Another advantage to retail pharmacies is they often offer extended hours, some 24 hours a day when you can fill your script (Costco is not 24 hours). Outside of that convenience, you should typically look at other pharmacy types.

Specialty pharmacies, much as the name implies, are focused mainly on dispensing specialty medications. What is a specialty medication you ask? These pharmaceuticals are high-cost, highly complex, and require high touch by a team of healthcare professionals. These drugs are often biologics, which means they are derived from living cells and are often injected or infused intravenously. However, more and more of these specialty drugs are offered in tablet or capsule form too. Due to the complexity of these medications, I have devoted an entire step (step 24) to them. It could make a difference in price where you go; however, in some cases, only certain pharmacies can fill these medications. The manufacturers give access only to those pharmacies that show that they can provide the specialized counseling and medication services needed when the drug is dispensed; services far beyond the typical dispensing a retail pharmacy would do.

Next on the list is mail order pharmacies. These are often tied in with the pharmacy benefit manager who administers your prescription benefits. If they have a mail order pharmacy, they will offer a discount for you filling through the mail for typically a larger supply, mostly pushing a 90-day supply. You should note the copay for mail order on your medication talking points. It is usually a part of your benefit, and you will not normally see these pharmacies offer cash prices like you can see with retail pharmacies using the sites we discussed previously. A few things to note are that if this ends up being your most economical route, you will want to try to get all your so-called maintenance meds (those you take on an ongoing basis) via mail order. You will want to provide time for the scripts to get to you, like when you order something from Amazon. This will take longer than Amazon Prime for delivery, sometimes up to a week, so be sure to keep that in mind. If you go the mail order route, ask your prescriber for a split script. The prescriber will send a script to the mail order pharmacy for a 90-day supply, and a script to the retail store with the best price for around a 14-day supply, so you have plenty of medication on hand while you wait for the mail to come. Use your price-checking app to make the decision on where the short script should go, or if you know your insurance copay, use whatever is the lowest price option. Once you get the mail order script, and assuming it has refills, make sure to set a reminder of some kind to be able to notify you to refill the med 2-3 weeks in advance of needing it. The mail order will likely give you an option to do automatic refills. BEWARE of this approach. You can easily end up with a cabinet full of medication and a large bill to pay. Another tip here, don't set up the auto pay on the credit card, they do this to suck you into automatic refills, and you do not have a chance to review the need for the med based on your journaling before you are charged again. If you are thinking of discontinuing the medication after talking to your doctor, you could be on the hook for another 90-day supply instead of just 30. As you can see, the costs could add up quickly.

Independent pharmacies are a good option overlooked by many people. Your independent pharmacy has the tough challenge of competing with the larger chains. They are often locally owned and operated. They will be staffed with pharmacists who are interested in finding and retaining customers; you will not be just a number. They often can purchase drugs at a very similar price to the large chains. In cases where you find a good price on one medication but not the others on your list, do not be afraid to ask them if they will price match. Many times, they will, and you can stay with a pharmacy that will cater to you. Typically, other services they provide are included, such as delivery or professional services like medication therapy management. Don't forget to negotiate with these pharmacies. Often, they will have more autonomy than a chain pharmacy to lower prices for you. This can be effective even for generic medications. Another important reason to use the power of negotiating with independent pharmacies is it prevents you from having polypharmacy. Polypharmacy is where you are getting meds from several different pharmacies. To save money you may not be able to avoid polypharmacy. The danger in polypharmacy is that the different pharmacists do not know about all the medications you are taking. We can mitigate this risk using your medication list, but if you can avoid polypharmacy by using an independent pharmacy that is convenient, that is what I call killing two birds with one stone.

Many online pharmacies exist, but they are not all equal. As with many things on the internet, you need to proceed with caution when looking at these sites. Don't be fooled by prices that seem too low to be true when compared to others. How do you confirm if the site you are dealing with is legitimate and safe? The FDA has safety tips for buying medicine and medical products online. The key is never pay a fee to get drugs at a discount! They are likely using discount programs that you don't know about to get the discount and profiting off you with the monthly or annual fee. National Association of Boards of Pharmacy (NABP) developed the Verified Internet Pharmacy Practice Sites (VIPPS) program in the spring of 1999. Look for sites that have a Verified Internet Pharmacy Practice Site (VIPPS) seal (see figure 15) from the National Association of Boards of Pharmacy or a ". pharmacy" address. Additionally, Pharmacychecker.com is a great online resource that has pharmacy ratings, profiles and drug-price comparisons right on their site. Another great resource is the FDA's BeSafeRx that can help you identify and avoid fake online pharmacies. Remember; never buy from an online pharmacy that doesn't require a prescription

Figure 15

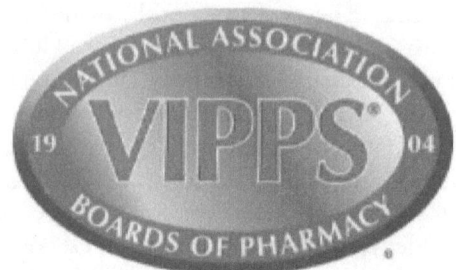

Some online pharmacies exist outside the U.S. and many are Canadian. In recent years, news headlines have discussed importing medications from Canada. If you find this as a good source to save on a medication on your medication talking points, then make sure the Canadian International Pharmacy Association (CIPA) has certified the online pharmacies. According to the National Library of Medicine, their review from 2013 of Canadian Price comparisons found the prices paid by patients for some common generics showed a higher price from Canadian pharmacies. The prices also did not take into consideration shipping charges from Canadian pharmacies, which can range from $20-30.

Certain states have also formed a cartel to buy prescription drugs from pharmacies in Ireland, Britain and Canada. The website Isaverx.net requires pharmacies abroad to meet those states safety rules set forth in that cartel. You should review this option with the FDA references, such as BeSafeRx, to ensure that all safety concerns are met.

Amazon is a much-hyped online resource for purchasing just about anything imaginable. However, at this point in time, you can't buy prescription medications on Amazon. However, they do sell many over the counter medications, herbal products, dietary supplements and a vast array of supplies. Recent headlines and the acquisition of a company called PillPack does make it seem like Amazon is trying to enter further into the pharmacy world, but right now they are limited to non-prescription only.

Another option for patients who have no insurance is a pharmacy called RxOutreach. This is used when all other options have been exhausted; you have looked for both free and $4 pharmacy generic programs, and you do not qualify for assistance programs (see step 20) or Medicare or Medicaid. RxOutreach does not require a coupon or a discount card. They only need your name, address or prescriber address, a prescription and the payment. They are a self-attestation pharmacy, and they don't require legal documents. They take a leap of faith that you have exhausted all other options. There is no paperwork, and they offer enrollment over the phone with a representative. Currently they have about 400 prescription products, so not all drugs will be available from this pharmacy. They mail the prescriptions to you and may be a good option when you have tried all the other items mentioned in this book.

Your medication talking points has different types of pharmacies listed. Using your insurance and the drug pricing tools that were mentioned, you should be able to indicate prices at the various pharmacy types to help you identify the ones that will offer you the greatest amount of savings.

Step 14: Check the Quantity

You need to pay attention to the quantity of medication your prescription is being written for; it could cost you if you don't. Pharmacies can't take medication back once they have dispensed it to you. They will have to destroy it if you don't use it. If the prescriber writes a prescription for a 30-day supply with 12 refills, you do not want to assume you will get all of that filled up front. If you are using insurance, and you have a copay that you can afford, then you will want to get the 30-day supply filled up front. However, if you are planning to pay cash, then it makes sense to only get as many as you and your doctor agree will give you an adequate trial. Let's say that you and your doctor decide that 2 weeks is a sufficient trial. You can take the script to the pharmacy and tell the pharmacist you only want 14 of the 30-day supply filled. They will then charge you the cash price for 14 days' worth. If you decide this medication is helping you, and you want to continue based on your notes in your journal, then you can go back and buy the remaining 16-day supply. The lesson here is you can get a partial fill of a script from your pharmacy. If the pharmacy says they won't do that, move on to the next one.

On the other hand, if you have a prescription for a medication that has proven benefits for you and long-term therapy is expected, you should take a different approach. You should identify the medications that fit that profile on your medication talking points. Like with many retail purchases, buying in bulk can often provide you a nice discount. You will have to ask the pharmacy for this, since pharmacies don't advertise this type of cost savings. So, look at the pharmacy who will provide the lowest price, and then ask if they offer a discount for bulk purchases. This tactic may require that you have your doctor write the prescription for a larger quantity, and you will need to coordinate that between the office and the pharmacy, but the discount could be worth the effort. Figure 16 lays out the savings power of buying in bulk for a generic medication, topiramate 25mg, which is used for migraine prevention and partial seizures.

Figure 16
Topiramate 25mg. Kroger pharmacy, source GoodRx
- 30 tabs $5.69
- 60 tabs $10.37
- 90 tabs $12.34
- 120 tabs $13.37
- 180 tabs $15.43

As you can see the cost per tablet when buying 30 tabs was $0.19, but when you buy 180 tabs, the cost per tab was reduced greatly to $0.08. That is a 68% savings! Definitely worth a few minutes of your time to coordinate. One thing to keep in mind is that if your medication is a controlled substance (meds closely monitored since, they have a high potential for abuse), you may have trouble getting those scripts in large quantities due to increased laws in effect for these medications. Your medication talking points has a reminder for you to investigate bulk quantity discounts. As mentioned earlier, you will need to confirm that you will use the medication chronically and that it is non-controlled. If both are true, the quantity discount can add up quickly.

Step 15: Tablet Splitting

Certain medications come in many different strengths. An example would be atorvastatin, the generic for the commonly used medication for cholesterol, Lipitor. Atorvastatin is available as 10mg, 20mg, 40mg, and 80mg tablets. However, the cost of the 80mg is not eight times the cost of the 10mg as you might expect. See the price comparisons for 30 tablets in Figure 17.

Figure 17:

Source GoodRx

Atorvastatin 10mg   *$10.88*
                20mg   *$9.19*
                40mg   *$9.60*
                80mg   *$10.35*

As you can see the price difference is minimal between the strengths. The thing to note is that you can easily split atorvastatin tablets with a pill splitter. If your dose is 20mg, and you buy the 40mg you essentially cut the cost by 50%. Therefore, you need to determine if you can split the tablets you are taking. Not all medications are safe to split. You should ask your pharmacist if the medications that you take could be split. Make sure to indicate this on your medication talking points and be ready to ask your doctor about writing for the higher strength and changing the directions to ½ tablet.

Another thing to think about when considering quantity for your medication talking points is to highlight medications that you take multiple times per day. These are good candidates for a discussion with your prescriber about if you really need multiple times per day, or if you can get by with taking the prescribed medicine once per day or even every other day. A commonly prescribed medication for blood pressure, amlodipine, brand name Norvasc, is only indicated for once per day dosing. However, I often see doctors putting patients on this medication twice per day when the blood pressure isn't controlled by the once per day dose. In this case, the patient could be more compliant and save cash by going with a higher strength of amlodipine once per day, while still getting the same clinical effect due to the long half-life the drug has in the body. For example, your doctor could prescribe amlodipine 10mg once per day instead of 5mg twice per day. Not all medications will have the same ability to reduce the number of times per day you take it, but it is worth the conversation.

Step 16: Combo Pills

Certain medications are often used together, some examples include those to treat high blood pressure, high cholesterol, diabetes, cough and cold and many other disease states. Drug manufacturers took note of the fact that the meds were used together, and they created new pills that contain both medications in one. The original reason the drug manufacturers did this was to have another brand name medication that they could charge higher prices for. However, at this point, many of these combination medications are past their patent dates and generics are now available. So now, you can take two medications on your medication talking points and reduce them down to one. Some combination medications have three medications in them, maybe more than that for cough and cold medications. How do you identify which combo pills are available, so you are ready for the conversation with your prescriber on this saving step? A google search of the name of the drug you take, and the words combination medication will give you an idea if a combination exists. You should check with your pharmacist if you can't find anything online. Mark down the potential options you have and prepare to save big.

A 2016 study in *The Journal of the American Medical Association* (JAMA) stated that Medicare Part D would have saved more than $925 million by using generic combination meds.[35] That is almost a billion dollars in savings just from this one method! They focused on 28 combination drugs of both brand and generic versions. Most of those drugs were used to treat cardiovascular disease. If you take medications to treat cardiovascular conditions, you must investigate combination products.

Combination pills can work the opposite way as well. If you are taking a brand name drug comprised of two or more drugs, you need to look and see if the individual components are available generically. In some cases, you will be able to achieve significant savings by using generic individual drugs. An example of this is Zegerid, which treats gastrointestinal problems. It is comprised of omeprazole and sodium bicarbonate. For a 30-day supply of Zegerid, you can expect to spend about $215, if you pay cash with no insurance. The cost of the generic components is roughly $15. This $200 per month savings quickly adds up to $2400 per year, just by looking into breaking up an expensive brand name combination drug.

Step 17: Dosage Forms

Does the drug you take have an extended release version? Metoprolol tartrate, generic for Lopressor, used to treat high blood pressure and control heart rate, is dosed 2-3 times per day. Another version of the drug, metoprolol succinate, generic for Toprol XL, was introduced. It typically has once per day dosing. Both forms are now available generically, so you might be able to get an easier to take, once per day medication vs twice per day, and save money in the process. You would need to discuss with your doctor or pharmacist if any of those opportunities exist for you. The key is to do your homework by scanning your medication list for drugs used multiple times per day.

Most medications used today and that we have talked about thus far are for some type of oral capsule or tablet. Not all medications are in the oral dosage form and often the non-oral products can be quite expensive, so how can you save on these mediations? Let's take a detailed look at the various forms available, and how you can save when using them.

Eye drops can be very costly, and you typically don't have very many options on package size or how big the bottle is. Therefore, it is hard to use our bulk quantity tricks in this area. Also, these medications do not follow the same quantity rules. They are just as expensive or maybe more expensive for a larger amount. So how do you save money on these prescriptions? According to an article in the *Medical Letter* from June 2006, researchers found that the eyeball can only hold about 10 microliters of fluid. A drop from an eye dropper delivers 25 to 50 microliters.[36] If you are using two drops (which I have seen regularly in practice) of an eye medication, the second drop is literally all waste and going right down your tear duct costing you a large amount of cash. On your next visit to see your prescriber ask them if they are aware of the amount of medication the eyeball can hold. If you take more than one drop of an eye medication, you might be able to reduce your dose to one drop. Also, make sure you hold down on your tear duct at the inside of your eyeball with your thumb or index finger for about 5 minutes after taking a drop, this will keep the medication in your eye longer, hopefully delivering maximum benefit to you.

Eardrops are another category of medication where you want to ensure you know how to use the medication correctly. Administering the medication in a way that will allow you to get maximum benefit from the smallest needed amount of the medication is key. You need to ensure you are getting the drops into the ear. If you are not able to do this by yourself, find someone who can help administer the drops for you. Holding your ear up and back, laying your head to the side, pressing on the skin over the ear after the drops are in to help it run down the ear canal, and possibly using cotton balls are some key points to prevent wasting the medication. Your pharmacist can give you full counseling on the administration of eardrops. Since ear medications are relatively uncommon in use, make sure the generic and therapeutic equivalents steps are used.

Nasal administration of certain medications can be a very effective way to deliver the drug where needed and to provide benefit with less likelihood of side effects. However, this formulation can come at a high price. Utilizing the medication to get maximum effect can save you money over time. Often you will see directions of 1-2 inhalations, and if you can get by with using one inhalation instead of two, then your bottle of nasal spray will indeed last longer and thus cost less over time. Some important counseling tips would be to blow your nose gently before use, which should allow for more absorption of the medication, keep your head upright, block off the other nostril, and breathe in quickly while squeezing the bottle. If you use these tips and journal on the medication's effect, you should be able to tell if you can have maximum benefit from one spray instead of two or more. As with ear drops you need to make sure to use the generic and therapeutic equivalent steps. Another good idea is to see if the medication you take is available over the counter. In some cases, this may save you money as well.

Creams and Ointments have multiple different strengths and forms of the same drug that affect potency. In general, steroid creams are broken out into low, medium, and high potency strengths. Your doctor probably does not care which drug you get specifically if you get one that is in a low, medium, or high potency. You can obtain big savings by checking on which form is going to cost the least. Work with your pharmacist to identify good options as your prescriber will likely not be aware of all the potential options by potency range. If the cream or ointment that you are prescribed does not contain steroids, a good option is to look at over the counter options for price savings. Knowing the size of the area you need to treat will be a key point also. If you have three small spots about the size of a fingertip on your leg to treat, then you do not need a large 60-gram tube. You might pay through the nose for the bigger tube when a small 15-gram tube would have lasted you through your course of therapy. Saving point: don't buy large quantities that you will ultimately end up throwing away.

Oral inhalers have caused pain to the pocketbooks of many Americans since 2009, the year when a new regulation went into effect that eliminated the old propellant called CFC's from use. Inhalers that had been generically available for some time were now being sold as new brands since the new HFA propellant made them new drugs in the eyes of the FDA. With so many brands and few generics available, how can you save money? First, you should know your disease. Your doctor most likely started you on a higher dose for these inhalers in the beginning due to the severity of your symptoms. Now your disease might be under better control, and your doctor could decrease your dose or possibly stop one of your medications. These are important things to note on your medication talking points if you use inhalers. Please note that these meds are never to be changed without discussing with your doctor first. Make sure you know which inhalers you take every day and which you should only use as needed. Many patients use their rescue inhalers too often and daily inhalers less than daily. This can have dire consequences. The important thing to remember with the disease states that require oral inhalers is the cost of going to the emergency room is much higher than the cost of getting your inhaler script filled. Nebulized solutions of medications such as albuterol might be a cheaper option than regularly filling scripts for inhalers. Nebulized inhalers do require a nebulizer machine, but that often delivers the medicine into your lungs more effectively than oral inhalers. Carrying an inhaler with you when you are away from home and using a nebulizer for home treatments could help lower your overall costs. If nebulizers are not an option, and you need to get an oral inhaler, then make sure you obtain a spacer. The spacer allows you to load the dose from the inhaler into the spacer. Getting the dose delivered into your lungs from the spacer is much easier than from the inhaler due to the dexterity it takes to inhale and administer the inhaler dose at the same time. You can save on inhalers by using the spacer because you can often get the desired effects with fewer inhalations utilizing the spacer.

Prescription for Maximum Savings

It may not sound like a lot but using two less inhalers per year can mean hundreds of dollars.

Step 18: Review Your Allergies and Intolerances

One of the most confusing parts of a medical chart is the list of patient allergies. Allergies are defined as a damaging immune response by the body to a substance, medication, food, pollen or dust, to which it has become hypersensitive. The most common allergic reactions that can result from using a medication include:

- Itching
- Hives
- Swelling of lips, face, tongue, limbs or throat
- Wheezing or nasal congestion
- Abdominal pain, diarrhea, nausea or vomiting
- Dizziness, or fainting

In some cases, if you took a medication and had one of these reactions immediately following, you could confirm the medication caused that reaction. Many times, however, the incident happened so long ago, that the true reaction may or may not have been related to the medicine. If you were in the hospital or sick, you may have been exposed to many new medications, so it is hard to confirm that one or the other caused the reaction. Sometimes the allergy comes from your mom or dad telling you that you can't use something because they were allergic to it. In addition, some medications list side effects such as nausea, but taking the medicine with food or following other pharmacy instructions can prevent these adverse effects. For the health of your pocketbook, you should not eliminate an effective and low-cost medication just because you think you have an allergy to it. It might be very mild or not an actual allergy at all. Please list all medications that you are allergic to on your medication talking points and see if those fall in a generic or therapeutic equivalent class that could save you money. IN ALL CASES, YOU MUST TALK TO YOUR DOCTOR FIRST. Certain reactions such as swelling of lips, face, tongue, limbs or throat are very serious and you should not retry that medication again.

When you see the ads for new prescription medications, you often hear a long list of side effects at the end. Do you really hear the side effect list or know what those conditions mean? They run through these quickly, but they are often significant. Always be suspicious of new side effects or allergies that appear after you start a new medication. Examples include rash, cough, sexual disorders, muscle aches, heartburn or depression. If the new medication is causing you to have a side effect, and you must get a second medication to treat the side effect from the first medication, that is a very expensive and inefficient process.

If you are truly allergic to a medication that your insurance prefers, and you must pay a much higher copay for a higher tiered alternative, you need to act as well. You will need to get your doctor involved to ask for an exception to take a brand name, non-preferred drug. This will require prior authorization paperwork and documentation from your doctor on your behalf. The process will take time, but it is worth the effort if there are no other options. You will be able to go from paying cash for a drug not covered or paying a non-preferred high copay to paying a preferred copay that will be much cheaper, especially for chronic therapy.

Step 19: Samples

Many internet resources that talk about how to save money on prescription drugs will talk about samples passed out from doctors on behalf of the drug manufacturer. You should be wary of thinking that samples are a good way to save money long term. The steps listed above will ensure you save money over the long run. Samples end up being a short-term solution only in certain circumstances. Think about what samples are: a marketing material, and not a means to an end. Once the samples run out, whether it is in two weeks or six months, they will run out, and when they do, you will be stuck with the high bill at the pharmacy counter. You will notice that the only drugs the doctor has samples of are the expensive Me-too drugs or new novel therapies that are very expensive. You will not see doctors passing out samples of generic medications because no drug company is going to put those in the sample locker for them to pass out to patients. A 2006 article published in the *Journal of the American Medical Association* showed that samples have a powerful effect on prescribers, causing them to use drugs that are more expensive but not necessarily more effective.[37] The other problem is that invariably the medications your doctor has samples of will not be on your formulary, unless you get lucky. What this means is the cash prices are going to be very high, therefore using your insurance will make sense, but a non-formulary drug is going to cost you more. Therefore, I came up with the following rules for you if you must use samples:

- Make sure you talk to your doctor about therapeutic equivalents first. (Step 12)

- If no therapeutic equivalent from Step 12 is available, then check your formulary for the class of medication you need to take. (Formulary research was explained in Step 7)

- What type of treatment is this? Short term like an antibiotic or longer term also known as a maintenance med. If short term, do they have samples for your whole course of therapy? If so, no further action needed take the samples. If longer term, see the steps below.

- Once you identify the formulary drug, ask for samples of that drug. Ask your doctor how long it would take to see the desired effect of the medication or to make sure no side effects occur. Ask for enough samples to get you through that trial period. It might take one month to try the medicine and come back to see your doctor at the next appointment. Remind the doctor you are trying to be economical about your prescriptions, and if the trial period can be shorter, you would like to know that. This serves two purposes; it saves you money and prevents you from taking longer than needed to get to an effective treatment for your condition.

- If they don't have enough samples to get you through the trial period, only purchase enough medication that when added to the samples will get you through the trial period.

- Make sure that your prescriber does not send a prescription to the pharmacy for an extended period, such as a 30, 60 or 90-day supply, until you have finished the trial and determined that it is the right medication for you. You might have to make an exception for specialty medications where you must wait for prior authorization or determine eligibility for a patient assistance program. See the specialty section for more details.

- Journal extensively from day 1 through the last day of your sample's trial so you can make an informed decision of whether you should get this medication or try something else.

- During the trial period, you need to see if a Patient Assistance Program or a state sponsored Patient Assistance Program exists, see step 20 & 21.

- If no Patient Assistance Program exists, check to see what manufacturer coupons or discount programs exist. See step 22 on manufacturer coupons.

- If you need medication via samples then stock up!

Step 20: Pharmaceutical Assistance Programs (PAP's)

Patient Assistance Programs (PAPs) are programs created by pharmaceutical manufacturers to help financially needy patients obtain necessary medications. The manufacturers set these up as nonprofit charitable organizations. Through these programs, medications are available at no cost or at a minimal fee. Many types of PAPs exist, including those for patients that do not have insurance, for individuals whose insurance copayment amounts are very expensive, and other programs to assist with specific types of insurance. These programs target patients with low and moderate incomes and older adults and those suffering with chronic conditions that require multiple medications and thus face the greatest need for these types of discounts. These uninsured or underinsured patients also tend to take less of their medication than has been prescribed due to cost concerns. Uninsured patients are twice as likely as insured to underuse their medications to lower drug costs, according to Center for Medicare and Medicaid Services. PAP's are funded through donations and thus do not continually have funding to keep the program open. You will need to confirm if funding is still available before you endeavor to enroll in the programs.

Specialty medications are increasing rapidly as a percentage of the overall drug spending. However, specialty brand and generic drugs can all have patient assistance programs of one type or another. More and more patients are exposed to higher cost sharing with complex drug therapies and high deductible health plans. This leads to a need for more assistance. Many manufacturers offer coupons and discounts, but that is NOT the first place you should look for assistance. More to come on manufacturer coupons in a following step. Most patients do not realize you should always look for pharmaceutical assistance programs (PAP's) first. These sometimes look like they are associated with pharmaceutical companies, but they are different as they set them up as charitable non-profit organizations. PAP's may be owned by one manufacturer, while others have multiple manufacturers come together to form a PAP, often associated with a disease state or other reason.

A study done by the Kaiser foundation in 2015 found that just over 1 million Medicare Part D enrollees reached the catastrophic coverage level which was more than double the 2007 number of 407,000.[38] Catastrophic coverage means they have exceeded the amount due in the coverage gap where you are responsible for the full cost of medications. For 2018 once you have spent $5,000 out of pocket, you are in the catastrophic range and you will only pay a small coinsurance or copayment for covered drugs the rest of the year. Most commercial insurance plans are set up in a similar fashion. This increasing trend of very high spending is expected to continue, and therefore you need to understand the key concepts in this step of the process. While enrolling in PAP's can be time consuming, it can be well worth it, considering the amount of savings that you could realize. Additionally, knowing the tricks will help you realize much faster if you will qualify for a PAP or if you should move to the next step.

All PAPs are designed to help those in need, and since different companies or groups of companies establish them, guidelines are all different. There are no laws governing PAP programs, so you only must meet eligibility requirements. In some cases, you must have insurance; and in other cases, you must not have insurance. Eligibility to participate in a PAP varies for patients with Medicare, but these must operate "outside the Part D benefit." Medicare beneficiaries who don't have supplemental drug coverage will be able to get assistance on a case-by-case basis, while others will deny assistance to those patients who are eligible for drug benefits from any public assistance program. That would include state and local programs. An important point to remember is that for Medicare Part D any assistance received would NOT count toward out of pocket expenses. Meaning the amounts would not apply toward deductible, initial coverage limit or catastrophic coverage. In most cases with Medicare, you must apply for other forms of public assistance before you can receive PAP funds, such as the Part D low-income subsidy if that applies to your situation. You can find more details on Medicare at www.cms.gov.

Keep in mind that CMS tracks who gets PAP funds. They have instituted data exchanges with the PAPs, including State PAPs, to help them coordinate the Medicare Part D drug benefit. That data exchange allows them to accurately pay claims through the program and calculate the true out of pocket expenses mentioned above. Therefore, you should not try to avoid accurately reporting this on taxes or other legal documents.

      The first thing to do is get the medication talking points and identify the drugs that need to be researched for PAPs. Remember this is not just for brand name medications. To find generics listed under PAP programs, you will need to search by disease state. Next, go to the NeedyMeds.org website and look under patient assistance for any PAP programs available for the drug(s) in question. NeedyMeds is a non-profit funded by donations and other sources. Once you find the drug, searching either by drug or by disease, you will see icons. If the PAP icon shows for your drug(s), then there is a PAP program available. Click on it and see what the eligibility requirements are. It will give you an income level as a percentage of the federal poverty limit (FPL). Don't despair; these limits are not just for people below the FPL! Some allow for up to 500% of the FPL, which is a good income. Eligibility will also be based on insurance status and family size. Needymeds has a calculator on their site that will calculate where you fall as a percentage of the FPL. You just must put in your income as reported on your tax documents the previous year and the number of people in your household reported on your tax records, then hit submit. It will give you your percentage of the FPL. For example, the program might require you be at or below 300% of the FPL. When you do the FPL calculator and find your income based on family size is 275% of FPL, you know you can qualify for the program, and you should discuss this with your prescriber if you fit the other criteria. In addition, if you come up at just above the FPL level for a given program, you should not just mark that program off. Rather you should contact the PAP and ask them to make an economic hardship request. These requests are often granted and definitely worth your time. The contact information is listed on the NeedyMeds site. Needymeds does not have a PAP program of its own but does have a drug discount card discussed in step 10. The best way to find out about these programs is via the web. If you don't have a computer, you can go to a public library or ask to use a friend or family member's computer. You will not actually be applying online, so your personal data will not be shared. You will just be printing off the application forms.

      Your doctor will need to be involved for you to be able to qualify, but you MUST do the research ahead of time to ensure you only discuss with your prescriber the programs you can enroll in. Remember your doctor is not the best resource for information on PAPs. In fact, they may not even know what they are. Pharmacists are likely to be more aware, but still will not be up to date on all programs that could help you. The best resource is to take the initiative yourself and complete this research. If you use the methods below, it will be much simpler. Once you complete your part, many will require only a doctor's signature, while some programs will require the prescriber complete a portion of the form as well. Below are some minimum requirements you should have ready before you make the appointment with your doctor to review your medication talking points.

- Print and complete the application form as best as you can prior to the appointment.

- Complete doctors' demographics for them (name, address phone number).

- Don't be surprised if the doctor doesn't fill out the forms immediately or has some office staff fill out the paperwork.

- If the doctor must fax information, then make sure you have all the appropriate documentation of income and any other items that only you would have for completion.

They will greatly appreciate the time you save them and will be more likely to help you with this process if you complete this pre-planning step. Your doctor may require a fee to complete this paperwork, and I would recommend you go ahead and pay for this service from your doctor because it is a valid request. Additionally, if your doctor has a social worker in the office, they may be a valuable resource to assist with this process. I have talked to patients who were upset because their doctor would not fill out PAP paperwork. If you do all the planning, pay the fee, and still cannot get your doctor to help you, then there are two things you should do.

1. Tell the doctor you will not be able to follow the therapy regimen they want for you due to the cost of the medication, and you want to work with them to improve your overall health.

2. If that still doesn't work, then you need to find a new doctor who will work with you on maximizing your savings on medications.

Citizenship may be a factor in eligibility criteria for PAPs. If the program says that you need to reside in the United States, then you will not have to provide documentation other than the fact you have resided in the U.S. This could be as simple as providing a bill with your name and present address on it. However, if it says citizenship, then you will need to provide documentation of citizenship. This might include a passport or other forms of identification.

PAP applications can seem overwhelming, especially if you must enroll in more than one program. There is help for this also. Needymeds.org has PAP application assistance programs that can be searched by zip code. Patient advocacy groups, HUB's and specialty pharmacies often offer completion services for enrollment forms as well. You provide them consent to use your information, and they will do the enrollment on your behalf for a fee. The HUB or specialty pharmacy may complete this free of charge as they have a financial incentive to see that you start the therapy. Keep this in mind before you pay for enrollment services. I am not saying that you can't complete these forms yourself, just letting you know that help is available. You must act on this step; the savings can be dramatic!

Several other resources in figure 18 are available to help you navigate PAP programs in addition to Needymeds. Most have websites that make it easy to find eligibility guidelines, how to enroll online, and links to other health resources. Many also offer toll-free telephone support. With so many websites available, it can almost be overwhelming, which is why I recommend you start with Needymeds. This will take some time but repeat this step using each of the sites below to ensure you don't miss a program for which you may qualify. From there you will need to search for the medication you use. You will also be able to look for help under the disease specific sections. If you can't find the medication by name, you can find the medication by looking up the disease for which your drug is prescribed. Next, complete the enrollment application, and based on how long you are on therapy you may have to re-enroll. The criteria may change over time, and your doctor will likely need to be involved.

After filling out the paperwork, it can take up to 4-6 weeks to hear if you qualify. These programs help support millions of patients and literally give away billions of dollars in assistance annually. Don't be in a hurry. Take your time, fill out forms completely, and ask for samples until the process is completed (Step 19). PAPs will distribute the medications in a variety of ways. Many will send the medication to the doctor's office, some to the pharmacy. Another method is to send you a certificate or card to take to the pharmacy to get your prescription filled. Most PAP programs will also provide assistance for refills of prescriptions for ongoing treatment of chronic diseases.

Figure 18

RxAssist	Web-based medication assistance resource center. Covers many issues related to medication access including low cost, Med D and PAP programs. Allows comparison of programs as well.
Partnership for Prescription Assistance Patient Services Inc. (PPA)	Sponsored by Pharma companies and helps qualifying patients get their medications. Many patients can get their medications free or nearly free. The patient assistance section of the website is where you get started.
Free Medicine Program	Helps patients obtain prescription drugs and medications free of charge. Established by volunteers and focused on patients with too much income to qualify for government prescription assistance programs but not enough to purchase private prescription drug insurance coverage, or who are living on retirement income, disability or other assistance. They do ask for a $5 donation for form submissions.
HHS	Department of Health & Human Services healthfinder.gov website offers insights from the FDA and other government agencies on numerous patient assistance programs for pharmaceuticals and other healthcare related items.
Pharmaceutical Research and Manufacturers of America (PhRMA)	An association and lobbying group, whose members include many of the larger pharmaceutical manufacturers, runs HelpingPatients.org, which has information on PhRMA members programs.

Another great resource on the NeedyMeds site is the diagnosis-based assistance. This can be your second greatest source of savings. They have a variety of savings opportunities on costs associated with the disease state, excluding the drug costs. This includes items such as medical supplies, equipment, testing strips, wigs, service animals etc. Some disease states such as diabetes are broken down into subcategories and the data can be searched by state. Two important columns to assist in research for these items are the services provided and areas of service. With a quick scan under the disease state you have, you can find all sorts of resources to lower costs and quickly decide if they are close to you.

With all the moving pieces involved in the PAP process, there will surely be questions that arise and here are some important considerations to keep in mind, so you don't get overwhelmed. If you get confused, remember your pharmacist is one of the best resources for you regarding the topics covered here. You ultimately want to go into the visit with your doctor with your medication talking points completed to the best of your ability. Your pharmacist will be able to help you fill in the gaps. Confide in your pharmacist about the cost of medications and tell them if you are not able to take your medication as prescribed due to costs. You will not be in trouble. They want the best outcome for your health, as does your doctor. You need a care team around you, and you can't be dependent on just one professional to get this all straight.

The methods described before have focused on patients who are insured or underinsured and, in some cases, uninsured. Patients with low income can also qualify for the Low-Income Subsidy (Extra Help) program. If you meet the requirements, your premiums will be reduced and deductibles for generics will be less than $3 and less than $8 for brands. The amount of premium subsidy is based on the amount of your countable resources. The criteria that need to be met includes:

- The patient is enrolled in both Medicare Parts A & B
- Patient resides in one of the 50 states or the District of Columbia
- Fall below the income and resource requirements

You do not need to be previously enrolled in a Medicare Part D Prescription Drug Plan (PDP) to enroll for Extra Help. If you do not meet these eligibility criteria, you may still be eligible for state assistance based on household size, earnings from work, or residency in Alaska or Hawaii.

Step 21: State Pharmaceutical Assistance Programs

What do you do if you have applied for a PAP program and you are not able to qualify because your income is too high or your out of pocket costs are not completely covered? The next step is to look at programs offered by individual states. Most states offer some form of Pharmaceutical Assistance Programs to help residents financially. State, county, or local governments fund these programs. They may administer the program or have a nonprofit institution. The programs provide not only prescription assistance but also insurance premium assistance; as well as help with medical supplies or equipment. Each of the programs works differently, and some will coordinate the program to work with Medicare Part D drug benefits. If you haven't signed up with Part D, but you are eligible, you may have to sign up to get your state benefit. In some cases, the state plans may help you pay for Medicare part D premiums as well.

An excellent guide to State health insurance assistance program websites (SPAP's) can be found by searching for Medicare.gov under State Pharmaceutical Assistance Programs. This site lists information on eligibility, contact numbers, addresses, links and other important notes. Some key points of these programs to keep in mind are that they kick in when other options have been exhausted, and they typically apply to low income elderly or disabled patients who do not qualify for Medicaid. They have restrictive formularies, so not every drug will be an option. Most programs charge a small copay, so this will not be completely free. Programs also exist that help with certain disease states specifically. These are coordinated with your Medicare Part D benefit. Not every state has the same programs, so you will need to verify the offerings in your state.

To provide you with easier processing of all these various programs, I would also refer you to Needymeds.org. Like PAP programs, Needymeds has a wealth of information on state PAP's also. You can either search under your state or look under Patient Assistance and then Government Programs for State Assistance. The programs are listed in alphabetical order once you select your state.

Most state laws enable these programs to be a Medicare adjunct benefit to fill gaps in coverage. Unlike what happens with commercial insurance, where coupons and some other forms of assistance do not count toward deductibles, state PAP's are different. When used with Medicare, these are considered as a portion of the true out of pocket expenses that you pay.

Step 22: Pharmaceutical Manufacturer Copay Coupons

Congratulations! You have made it deep into the step-by-step process to save money on prescription medications. If you are still looking for savings, you are sure to have already substantially improved your medication cost profile by this point. The next step involved is to look for manufacturer coupons. As I have spent many chapters steering you away from expensive brand name drugs, you can see why this comes as one of the last steps. Many patients who don't take the time to read a book like this will jump right in with a manufacturer coupon and then stop when searching for savings. They think, "Hey this is easy, and I saved a bunch!" Like many things in life if it seems too good to be true, it often is. Let me explain why.

What is a copay coupon? These coupons are offered to eligible patients to help reduce out of pocket costs, typically assisting with large copays or high deductibles. They can be used at almost any pharmacy. Patients with commercial insurance (non-Medicare/Medicaid or other federal or state healthcare insurance) can use them. Drug manufacturers typically give these coupons out to encourage you to use their brand name drug over a generic or therapeutic equivalent that would be much less expensive. The first problem is that not everyone is eligible to use these coupons. To prevent pharmaceutical manufacturers from trying to drive Medicare and Medicaid members toward their drug, the government has made those on government insurance programs ineligible for coupons. Coupons will allow you to fill the drug but only for a limited number of refills. This can cause problems for ongoing maintenance therapy for chronic diseases when you suddenly go from a $5 copay to paying a $500 bill 6 or 12 months later for the same medication. Keep in mind that manufacturers will be tracking information you provide them when you apply for these programs as well. This is something to keep in mind if your health information privacy is a concern for you.

According to data from IQVIA formulary impact analyzer, the use of coupon programs has increased rapidly.[39] Utilization went from 12% in 2013 to 18% in 2017. Additionally, the amount of average payment by the coupon cards has increased from $52 in 2013 to $93 in 2017. As you can see, these continue to play a bigger role in helping offset high copay, coinsurance and deductibles.

Due to this increased utilization, more insurance companies and Pharmacy Benefit Managers are implementing copay accumulators, which track how much money in manufacturer payments apply toward the patient's copay or coinsurance and making sure those amounts are not applied toward the patient's deductible or out of pocket maximum. This saves drug plans and insurers money by shifting payment to patients. Let's say you have a $5000 high deductible health plan, and you take a medication that costs $1500 per month. You were able to find a manufacturer coupon that pays $1500 per month for the first three months toward your copay. Normally after four months you would have to pay $500 to meet your deductible ($1500 x 3 months = $4500) + $500 out of your pocket = $5000 total deductible paid. However, with a copay accumulator program in place, the $4500 from the manufacturer would not apply. Meaning in month four, you are on the hook for the full $1500 (the price of the drug that month) not just $500, and still have $3500 more to go to meet your deductible. Will you be able to continue obtaining your medication from the pharmacy?

This is the reality more and more patients are facing when dealing with copay accumulators. The net result is that patients often quit taking the medication after they have been on it for a few months. The resulting non-adherence to therapy often ends up costing the plan and patient once they end up in the hospital or worse.

According to an NBGH survey of about 140 multistate employers with at least 5,000 workers, 17 percent reported they have a copay accumulator program in place this year.[40] They also found that 56 percent reported they're considering them for 2019 or 2020. An Xcenda Managed Care Network Survey in 2017 found over 80% of health plans and PBMs reported they were somewhat likely to limit copay assistance in the next two years.[41] As you can see, this is a growing problem that patients need to speak out on and understand what is occurring in their benefit design. You need to look for this when you are investigating the health plan you will select, especially if you take a medication and receive copay assistance.

Before you decide to pull the trigger on using a manufacturer coupon, you will need to review some research you did in Step 7. Find out if the drug is on your insurance's formulary or not. If it is, what copay tier is it in? You could find yourself in a situation where there are no generics or therapeutic alternative, but there is more than one branded drug available. If you had to pick a coupon program, you should do so for the one that is the most formulary preferred by your insurance. This is of course for those not covered by Medicare or Medicaid as coupons will not able allowed for those patients. Savings for you by finding the lowest cost copay using your insurance seems like a great plan; however, you need to remember that the drug company is not giving your insurance a discount. Your insurance is still paying that high brand price. Imagine if you have a $50 copay each month but use a coupon to get the cost down to $5 per month. Your insurer might still be paying $500 per month for that drug, and they do not get a coupon. Why should you care? If every patient using your insurance were to do this, you can imagine that the next year's premiums would have to rise in order to pay for all those pricey brand name medications. Thus, even though the coupon may seem like a great deal for you at the time, you must think about the long term, and how it can affect your premiums. You also need to keep in mind that if you do not have insurance, you may not be able to use a coupon. These programs are set up to be a form of secondary insurance, and if there is no primary insurance, often the process will not work. If you don't have insurance, be sure to ask if you are eligible before you apply for the coupon card.

The trend towards high deductible health plans has made the prevalence of coupon programs increase. Patients with large copays or deductibles often need assistance with those cash outlays. This has increased the number of programs also, so be aware of scams. Do not pay to get access to a coupon! Manufacturers will not require you to pay for a coupon for reasons described above, and a pharmacy may not even accept the paid coupon programs.

To apply for a manufacturer coupon, you will need to search online. The simplest way to locate the program is to google the name of the drug followed by the word coupon. You can also search on sites such as NeedyMeds.org under coupons. When applying, provide your demographic information, diagnosis, medication name, insurance information, your income and the number of people in your household.

Your doctor or pharmacist can complete the application, but most coupon programs will have simple requirements that you can complete. Once you have enrolled, you will receive a copay card, either electronically or via the mail. However, you are often eligible right after enrollment, so write down your information after you have completed the online enrollment, and you can use this information at the pharmacy until you receive your card. Some programs will have you pay for the script prior to getting your card, and then they will reimburse you after you have successfully enrolled. Most of the programs will provide you eligibility for 12 months because the program will want to confirm that you have insurance each year. At the end of each year, you will just need to reapply.

The final thing to keep in mind is that if you are having trouble affording your medication and the coupon runs out from the manufacturer, you can ask for an exception from the manufacturer. The key is to let the manufacturer know that you can't afford the medication without the coupon assistance, and that you will have to change your treatment to a less effective drug or become non-adherent to your medication without assistance. I am not saying you should lie about this. However, the cold hard truth is that many people are in this very situation today. What they need to know is that asking for this exception can keep the assistance coming.

Step 23: Expiration Dates

C edications you take on an as needed basis, and you are t with a small amount when you no longer need them. Perhaps you stopped a medication and had a large amount of excess that set in your medication cabinet. Later you find yourself needing to use that script again. Ever take a medication out of the cabinet, happy that you found them, only to realize the bottle says the medication expired 6 months ago? Does that expiration date mean you can't use the medication?

Drug expiration dates reflect the time during which the product is known to remain stable, retaining its strength and purity when stored appropriately. The potency of the drug must be between 90% to 110% of the strength on the medication label at the time the product is created. The expiration date is the date when the manufacturer or pharmacy who is repackaging the drug states that the drug will still meet the 90% potency of the original strength set forth by the FDA for labeled drugs. Thus, the expiration date doesn't mean the drug is necessarily bad or unable to be used, but rather that the manufacturer can't be sure that it is still 90% of the labeled potency, assuming it has been stored in appropriate conditions.

The date on a pill bottle is not the medication's true expiration date. The pharmacy puts a one-year expiration on all medications they take from the manufacturer's container and place into your individual bottle. Therefore, the expiration date you see will be sooner than when the drug actually expires. In some cases, several years might be cut off the actual life of the drug due to this practice. The pharmacy legally can't make it any longer than a year because no prescription is valid for longer than a year per FDA guidelines. This is because they want you to be in contact with your prescriber on at least a yearly basis, so you are routinely reevaluated. Knowing this can help you feel more confident about having a conversation with your doctor or pharmacist about medications you still have in your medicine cabinet. If you need to continue the drug, you might not need to throw those pills out. Solid dosage forms such as tablets and capsules are the primary candidates to ask your doctor or pharmacist if it is safe to use past the expiration date. While it may be safe to take certain medications, you should always confirm before proceeding.

Some medications if not stored in appropriate conditions may have degraded and could potentially yield toxic compounds. Patients with serious life-threatening disease states may be at an increased risk from medications that were not stored properly. You should discard any drug not stored in proper conditions within the expiration date or any drug outside of the expiration date. There are a few other instances when using medications past their expiration date is not a good idea. Any medication that is not in a tablet or capsule form is probably not a good candidate for use past expiration. Examples include liquids, suspensions, some antibiotics, nitroglycerin, insulins, injections, creams, ointments, eye drops, or ear drops to name a few. These types of products could have contamination with bacteria or mold and should be avoided when past the expiration date. Remember this is not going to be a primary way to save on prescriptions year after year, so don't push the issue, your safety is always paramount

Step 24: Specialty Pharmacy and Biosimilars

The definition of a specialty pharmacy is a distribution channel for specialty drugs that are either high cost, high complexity and/or high touch. The complexity has to do with the handling and administration of the drug in either preparing it for use or distributing it. High touch refers to special requirements for labs, prior authorization, skilled nursing or pharmacy follow-ups, etc. after administering the drug. Specialty medications are grabbing more and more headlines. This is not really a surprise given the substantial cost of these medications. The latest figures show that specialty medications make up about 1% of all prescription claims but represent 37% of drug spending. Projections show that by 2020 the spending number will increase to 50% of all the money spent on drugs![43] The average cost for a specialty medication is typically more than $3,000 per prescription. Just one specialty medication can more than offset the gains you've made by following the multiple other steps in this process.

Aside from the cost, the diagnosis is often new for the patient, leading to stress and anxiety from the significant change the disease state may have on his/her life. Taking time to let the diagnosis sink in is required to aid in making financial decisions that are sound. Acting on impulse and emotion will result in overpayment on medications. You will need to review several variables. Does the treatment substantially improve outcomes? An example would be the high cost treatments for Hepatitis C. They are likely well worth the cost, as they can provide a cure for the disease in a short time. Is the specialty treatment markedly better than other treatment options? For instance, let's look at rheumatoid arthritis treatments that are new biologics vs older conventional treatments referred to as disease modifying antirheumatic drugs (DMARD's). Will the cost of the new biologic agent really yield that much more improvement over the conventional treatments? Is a 3% improvement in outcome, based on a questionnaire that has you rate your ability to move without pain, worth the additional cost of the medication? I am not saying the newer biologic treatments do not yield great results, because sometimes they do. However, you need to have a conversation with your doctor about the treatment guidelines for the disease state in question. Most major disease states have treatment guidelines published by certain groups specifically focused on that disease state, or by major medical groups. These guidelines are compiled by looking at all the data from clinical trials and studies done after the drug is on the market. Following these guidelines will be the way to get the most bang for your buck. Some might think this is a one size fits all approach, but don't be fooled. The guidelines consider certain factors that one patient may have, and another may not, so it can be individualized. These guidelines will act as a template that, together with your doctor and care team, you can use to build your best treatment plan that is both clinically and financially responsible.

    These specialty pharmacy medications are all brand name drugs. There are no generics! The cost saving measure to implement if you are taking a specialty medication is to find out if there is a biosimilar. The first biosimilar was approved in the United States in 2015. Biosimilars are an almost identical copy of the original product that is manufactured by a different company, like generics but different in a few important ways. Biologic drugs are very large and complex molecules that may consist of proteins formed from amino acids, often in a biological animal cell, thus the name biologics. Most biologics attach to or replace naturally occurring proteins in our body that are causing a problem, leading to the disease. Due to the size and complexity of these molecules, exact replicas can't be produced except by the company who made the original product using the exact same recipe and formula over and over. Since these are made by living cells, the production can take months and must be controlled very carefully. Due to the intense process required even to make a similar drug to the original, these biosimilars are still expensive to produce in their own right. The FDA approves biosimilars differently than they do small molecule generic drugs due to these differences. Today most biosimilars are approved as highly similar to its reference biologic product. They are also expected to have similar efficacy and safety to that reference product. Ultimately, what you need to know is that your pharmacist can't just switch you to a biosimilar like they can for a small molecule generic pill.

Therefore, when discussing specialty medications with your doctor, you need to have facts ahead of time about what if any biosimilars are available. If a biosimilar is available, does your doctor feel it is appropriate to switch you to that biosimilar?

Many studies have been published by reputable journals showing that switching to biosimilars is a safe and effective way to save money.[44] Much more data exists from European research because they have been using biosimilars since 2006. The first biosimilar was not approved in the United States until 2014. The most common concern with these interchanges to a biosimilar is something called immunogenicity. What is that? It is the concern that since these products are large protein molecules that your immune system might react to the drug causing you to feel ill and possibly cause damage to your own tissues. Switching from one product and then back to the other product is the biggest concern for immunogenicity. The thought is that you do not want to become immune to the drug used to treat your disease. In most cases, this risk of immunogenicity is low, but you should make sure to review this topic with your doctor and health care team when considering using a biosimilar. Remind your doctor that more data exists from European studies on immunogenicity than what is available from the FDA.

An estimate by one of the large PBM's, Express Scripts, suggests that biosimilars could save $250 billion in the next 10 years.[45] Savings from switching to a biosimilar can be substantial, especially if you are enrolled in a high deductible plan. Savings by switching could be in the thousands of dollars per year, and if you continue the therapy long term, tens of thousands. The pipeline is full of new biologic originator products (the new brand names) as well as biosimilars. The FDA has recently taken strides to speed the process for approval of biosimilars. This is great news as it will help drive down prices through competition in the marketplace. It is estimated that there are nearly $100 billion worth of biologics that will be coming off patent in the near future. If there are no biosimilars available for the specialty drug you take, make sure you keep checking back to gain these large savings.

Another component of specialty drug savings lies in how your insurance bills these drugs. Many patients realize that you have both medical and pharmacy benefits under most insurance plans. What they don't often realize is that the medical part of your insurance may in fact be a better option to have your specialty drug filled / billed under. For Medicare these are known as part B, which covers medical costs, and part D, which covers prescription drugs. A recent study from Avalere Health highlights that drug costs can vary greatly based on which portion of the benefit, pharmacy or medical is used. The use of supplemental health insurance policies allow the member to avoid paying large out of pocket costs when using the medical benefit. In fact, the Avalere study found that in 2016, out of pocket costs were about 33% higher for new cancer therapies covered under Part D than for those covered under Part B. That 33% was an $800 difference! Not every drug is a candidate for switching to the Medical benefit, as they usually must be infusions administered in the doctor's office or outpatient setting. For both your medical and pharmacy benefit, you should be aware of what your out of pocket maximums are and keep that in mind. Many new specialty therapies could easily cause you to meet the out of pocket max. If there is a substantial difference between the pharmacy and medical benefit, this could have a dramatic impact on your finances.

The International Federation of Health plans estimates that Americans pay from two to six times more than the rest of the world for brand name medications.[46] These high prices have led to a trend called Medical tourism. Medical tourism is defined as people who live in one country but travel to another country to receive medical care. In addition to surgical procedures, which had been the majority of medical tourism, we are now seeing this spill over into specialty medications also. Certain disease states such as cancer or rheumatoid arthritis could provide large savings even when travel is included. Imagine you were receiving a cancer treatment that was going to cost $50,000 to $60,000 for your treatment course, but you could receive the same treatment overseas for $10,000-$20,000. You can see that with those large numbers, the costs of an overseas flight don't seem too outrageous.

Once you get the financial components of getting your specialty script filled, you have a few other things to keep in mind. Specialty medications can take a substantial amount of time for prior authorizations and approvals to take place between healthcare providers, insurers, Pharmacy Benefit Managers, regulatory agencies and specialty pharmacies. The process can take between 3-6 weeks to get the actual medication depending on the workflow of your doctor. As specialty pharmacy have grown, the challenges in the process have become more complex and include:

- High administrative workload for staff members
- Insurance coverage issues
- Slow, poor communication with payers, pharmacies, etc.

This results in delays in patients starting or refilling critical medication. If you have already started on a specialty medication, don't just assume the refill can be processed quickly. Give at least a two-week notice to your pharmacy of needing a refill prior to running out of your medication. This is critically important to ensure you don't end up having a gap in therapy that could have potential harmful health effects. One thing that normally slows the process down for new prescriptions is getting patient consent and financial information. You should ensure that you provide your doctor's office with consent before you leave the office. Others may need consent as well such as the specialty pharmacy. You need to make sure you provide your contact information to your doctor and the pharmacy that will be filling your script, so they can contact you to get this consent when needed.

The financial information required often has to do with income, assets in some cases and family members in your household. Once you know you will be on a specialty medication, you will want to get this information together and ensure it matches what was on your previous tax returns. Having this quickly available will prevent further delays in the process if you must call the pharmacy back.

Your specialty pharmacy may provide contact information for organizations that can offer support for you and your family. In addition to support, these organizations provide educational information, along with resources for local, regional, and national organizations. If your specialty pharmacy doesn't have helpful tools, another good place to start gathering information is NeedyMeds.org. You can search by drug or diagnosis for discounts, coupons and patient assistance programs, which have been reviewed previously in this book. The diagnosis section also has resources for other ancillary services such as travel arrangements, medical equipment and even service animals that may be required for the disease state. Keep these other things in mind because the costs can add up quickly when added to the cost of the drug itself.

A final point to reiterate here is that specialty medications alone can blow your entire medication budget out of the water with just one drug. If you find yourself taking one of these medications, it is imperative that you monitor closely how it is working. This requires the journaling discussed previously in this book. Prior to starting therapy, discuss with your doctor or pharmacist exactly what effects the drug should have. Also, find out what typical side affects you should watch out for, what "normal" responses to the medication you should see, and over what period of time. If possible, start journaling prior to starting the medication, so you can see a true before and after of your symptoms. You may also try having someone video your range of motion or the lesion on your skin prior to and after therapy, so you can compare before to after. In certain cases, you will not be able to tell if you feel better because the outcome is to improve a lab marker of some kind. In those cases, you still must journal to ensure that the side effects don't outweigh the benefit of the drug. If you don't see improvements as expected in the timeframe that you and your doctor were expecting, seek other options, maybe older more conventional medication therapies combined with non-medication treatments. It might be that you change from one specialty medication to another to see better results. The moral of the story is if you don't journal, you don't know if you feel better. If you don't feel better, and you are spending thousands of dollars a year, then you are losing on both fronts. Don't be reluctant to talk to your doctor because you think you don't have any options. You do. If you have information to back up your argument, which would be the data in your journal, you always have options that can help reduce the cost of the medication for the disease state.

Step 25: Keeping it All Straight--Technology Tools

Today the options for tools to help you track your health are growing rapidly, especially on mobile platforms. A few pioneers in this area were websites such as Microsoft with the personal HealthVault, created in 2007, and Google's Google Health, created in 2008 and discontinued in 2011. Both were advanced for the time, and none of the patients knew quite what to do with the data. Doctors and health systems were afraid to share data due to privacy concerns as well. Now apps for mobile devices are making another push and starting to get some traction.

The leader at this point in time is the Apple Health App. It tracks a variety of data points, including nutritional information, physical activity levels, body temperature, blood pressure, glucose and more. If you use the Health Record component, and your insurer or doctor uses Health Records, it will allow you to import your medication list from your doctor's Electronic Medical Record (EMR). If they participate, your procedures, lab results, vaccination records and much more will be available as well. If you are not able to access the information from your prescriber's records, you can add in medications manually.

Cleveland Clinic recently announced that its patients now have access to their personal health information on their iPhones with the Health Records feature. They use Apple Health together with Epic EMR and the MyChart app, which offers patients a more comprehensive mobile access to their own health information. Apple Health Records also launched initiatives with 39 large health systems earlier in 2018. Many other sites have also been making this type of access to your medical records a reality. As I discussed previously, the key to bringing down prices of medications and medical care is to make everyone a conscientious consumer of healthcare. As the technology continues to evolve, it will help to arm you with information and make you a better consumer. Don't overlook these tools in your quest to lower your out of pocket expenses. As we move to a world where you have better access to health information, can better organize it, and seamlessly share it with other healthcare providers, less inefficiency will remain, and medical errors should drop. The apps will enable patients to track important values and make decisions on medication savings easier.

Numerous other apps exist for Android and other mobile phone platforms. The easiest way to stay connected with your medications via technology is to ask your doctor what options exist within their electronic medical record. If you are tech savvy and interested in having these features, using a mobile app will allow you to track this data on your mobile device, which can come in very handy. Start with free apps that have good reviews to see what you like and dislike. Once you feel comfortable with tracking the information in this way, you can opt to spend a few bucks on an app if you think it makes sense for you.

Another option is a patient portal. What is a patient portal you ask? It is a secure, online website used by your doctor's office to give their patients access to personal health information. You would need to enter a username and password much like with your email. After that is setup, you can access recent visits, doctor notes, medications, immunizations, allergies and lab results, to name a few things. Many portals also allow you to schedule appointments, make payments, message your doctor's office, and request refills as well. Most patient portals will have apps that make it easy to use on a mobile device. This type of technology is the way you will interact with your health care team in the future.

Step 26: Repeat this Process Each Year!

Your quest for savings is an ongoing journey. As you age, the likelihood of acquiring a disease that will require a medication increases. According to the American Association of Consultant Pharmacists, patients 65-69 take an average of 15 prescriptions per year, and those age 80-84 take an average of 18![42] That being said, you must not think that you perform this exercise once and forget it. If you are like most people prior to reading this book, you probably never looked at how much you spent on medication each year. You knew it was a lot but did not know the actual number. It was painful enough each month that you sought out ways to lower costs, which lead you here. The question is," What will you do now?" Will you take the knowledge of what you are spending now, take off how much you can save, and then include that as a line item in your monthly budget? After you have taken the time to walk through this step-by-step process the first time and lower your medication costs as much as possible, your budget will get a big boost. However, don't be fooled into thinking your medication costs might not climb again over time. The first time you go through this exercise will be the hardest but following up the next year will be much easier. Just like anything in your life that you organize and plan out, certain road bumps will arise. You might start a new medication mid-year, and while that is not ideal, it can easily be managed by looking at the steps and figuring out which are appropriate for that new medication. Every year your insurance is likely to change. You may have a completely new plan or the same plan but a different drug formulary. Understand that these changes could alter your strategy from year to year. Save your medication talking points documentation, so you can easily update the plan as these changes arise.

  Each year, typically in October, you will have to enroll in your insurance for the upcoming year. Any new medication additions or changes you have made could have an impact on the type of health insurance plan you should purchase. Many health insurance advisors can assist with the process of looking for a plan but be wary of sales representatives who are just trying to sell you a policy that will render them a high commission. Make sure they are willing to take the time to review your medication list and medication talking points. As you head into your next plan year, don't wait until your enrollment period starts to begin this review. If you can, look at your health plan options before the enrollment period. If you can't review the plans ahead of time, make sure you get on this task as soon as open enrollment begins, so you have ample time to review, compare and weigh your options. In most cases, you have only two weeks to enroll, so getting the review done early can provide for big savings opportunities. Given that many plans now come with a high deductible, they will also have a Health Savings Account (HSA). This account will be a way for you to save tax-free money to provide for medical and medication expenses.

  Your financial life should contain a team of professionals that can help you with taxes, insurance, finances, legal issue etc. The same is true for healthcare. You need to assemble a team consisting of a doctor, specialist, pharmacist, and nurses. While those seem obvious, some other professionals are required as well. If you are purchasing Medicare, a licensed insurance sales representative can help with decisions around the best cost saving plan for you to select. If you enroll into an employer plan, take the time to use the resources they offer to help you make the best decision. Remember you are stuck with the decision for the next year so choose wisely.

  That HSA has investment opportunities that you need to explore as well. This is where I would urge you to plan to talk about your medications and medical care with your financial planner. A registered investment advisor who acts as a fiduciary not just a sales representative is a critical team member to ensure your overall financial success in life. Given the impact that medication and medicine can have on your finances, it is of the utmost importance to have the HSA and the percentage of your income you spend on healthcare to be included in the calculations the financial advisor makes for you. Without this, you could severely underestimate how much money you will be spending on healthcare in retirement. The investments in the HSA itself need consideration of whether they will be invested for long-term or short-term purposes based on when you think you will need to use the money in the HSA. You can deposit up to $6700 per year for a family into an HSA, and those over 55 can do a catch-up contribution of $1000 in addition. A triple tax savings along with high contribution limits make an HSA a very effective option to save for future healthcare expenses. It should not be invested in the same way as your other retirement money. Please, pull in this member from your healthcare team and have that conversation on medication spending so you don't underestimate costs.

Women especially should review the medication talking points each year. Why is this more important for women? Women have a longer life expectancy than men do and over time will have more prescription usage on average than men. The old saying is that "men die; women breakdown," and thus they expend more dollars on healthcare. Women need to make sure they know what their financial situation is and where dollars are being spent and saved. As women age, and if their spouse passes away, it is a good idea to have a trusted younger adult to serve as the executor of not only their financial matters but also healthcare. Having someone who is familiar with your medications and health conditions can be vital if a hospital or nursing home stay happens. That person can help champion the prescription list and make sure that wires aren't crossed as they transition from one healthcare entity to another and back to home.

When getting ready to enroll for your health insurance make sure you do so with your medication in mind. Having your medication talking points handy will be of the utmost importance. As soon are you are able to review your open enrollment insurance options, you need to start doing so. You will have options that have a high deductible plan vs. a more standard plan. The difference being that the premiums, or what you pay each month, will be lower for the high deductible plan. The standard plans will have higher premiums but potentially less out of pocket total expenses.

You need to take your list of medications and add up the annual costs that you figured out when we did your medication talking points. Will those same medications be on your plans formulary next year, or will they be excluded, leaving you to pay a higher copay or worse yet having to cover the full cost? You should be able to view a list of drugs that are on and off formulary for the insurer that you are choosing for the next plan year. This will be important as you do your comparison.

The next thing to think about is will those cash or coupon deals be able to apply toward your deductible? Your deductible is the limit where you stop paying full price and have some sort of copay or coinsurance kick in. This will typically be the case until you reach your out of pocket maximum. Unfortunately, if you use cash pay or coupon type of programs, you may find your insurance doesn't always let you apply this toward your deductible. You should always ask your insurer to reimburse you for your out of pocket costs if you have a flexible spending account and/or apply them toward your deductible amount. The insurance company can consider your paying with a coupon or cash process as out of network. The key step is to remember to keep your receipts for everything that you buy not using your insurance. Then make sure to fill out the prescription reimbursement form from your insurer and mail, fax or electronically submit the form and your receipts to your insurer. Always make sure you save copies of everything submitted. If you have a high-deductible plan, and the scripts you pay for out of pocket are not applied to this, then you should evaluate the plan you select for the next year. Determine if it makes sense to continue to pay out of pocket instead of using the insurance. If you only have high deductible plan options, then as mentioned before, you should look at the insurance as only being used for serious medical issues. Often the savings on your premiums and paying out of pocket for discounted scripts is a bigger savings than buying a more inclusive plan with higher monthly premiums.

Once you meet your deductible, you will typically have some other type of coinsurance to pay until you spend your out of pocket maximum or the year ends before you reach that limit. If you fall into this category, an evaluation of the high deductible plan vs a standard more inclusive plan is going to be required. One other variable to keep in mind is the Health Savings Account (HSA) that goes along with high deductible plans. Many times, your insurer will give you money to put into this account to offset medical and prescription costs. This should factor into your decision on what health plan works best for you since the HSA can help you pay your deductible when needed and increase your healthcare savings by using pre-tax dollars.

Final thoughts

America has a problem with our outlook on healthcare today. With all the conveniences of modern society, we don't want to have to wait for a solution to a problem. We want instant gratification. That type of expectation was born from being the most advanced society in the history of the world, which has also come with its share of problems. When it comes to our health, we often think there is some magic pill to solve our health problem. In many cases, medical advances have made tremendous strides to improve quality and quantity of life. However, often we turn to medications when simple lifestyle changes would be the best remedy. Pharmaceutical manufacturers run direct to consumer ads making it appear that they can be our easy button fix to the ailment. Just take our pill and your problem will be gone. Well it isn't that simple, nor is it safe for your wallet, or your long-term health. The problem is large with many players involved and much blame to go around.

You have now taken the time to read this book all the way to the end. Congratulations on making it past that hurdle! Now you have put yourself in the minority who acknowledges there is a problem, invests time and money in learning how to overcome it, and reads the material. The next step is the most important one in this step-by-step guide, as it is for anything in life. Take action! You may not be able to get through all the steps in this guide today but take a small step today that will move you on toward your goal of saving money on prescription medications. In the words of the legendary motivational speaker, Zig Ziglar, "Take as big a step as you can, but do it TODAY, that is the key!"

You might be able to save a few dollars here and there by jumping in at a step in the middle of the guide and feeling that you have done something. No doubt you have, but I would hate to see you short change what you could do to save money and improve your overall health. All prescription medications come with risks in addition to the benefits. Missing out on journaling and drug discontinuation conversations with your doctor could lead to poorer outcomes for your health. In this book, I have given you proven methods to save money and eliminate unneeded medication use. As a practicing pharmacist for over 15 years, I have seen medication prescribed with little or no thought given to the financial implications. I felt compelled to offer a solution that can prevent this, which is why I wrote this book. The step-by-step process to maximize your savings on your healthcare dollars will work for you and your family.

So, what happens now? You have read the steps, so you know how to save the most you can. Your medication appointment with your doctor should be getting close. You should have all your pre-visit homework complete at this point. Imagine how good it is going to feel when you walk out of the doctor's office knowing you are in control of your medication spending and your overall health. Tell your spouse, children, and friends about the changes you are making to help trigger conversations about this in the future. Help spread the word that everyone can take control of their health and lower their medication spending with this multi-step process!

Appendix A

- Appeal- the action you can take if you or your doctor disagree with a coverage decision made by your health plan. Appeals can be for the amount of the drug you get or how much you pay in some cases.
- Beneficiary- The person who has the health care insurance.
- Claim- a request for payment that you or your pharmacy submits to your health insurance when you get medications or devices that you think are covered.
- Coinsurance- amount you may be required to pay as your share of the cost of a medication or device after you pay any deductibles. Coinsurance is usually a percentage (example 25%)
- Coordination of benefits- a way to figure out who pays first when 2 or more health insurance plans are responsible for paying the same medical claim. You also may hear this term for the required paperwork your insurance must send to you after a medical procedure has taken place. Often you will receive these for pharmacy services on a quarterly basis.
- Copay - the amount you may be required to pay as your share of the cost for a medication, service or device. A copayment is normally a set amount instead of a percentage like coinsurance. For example, you may have a $10 copay for generics and a $50 copay for brand medications.
- Cost sharing - the amount you may be required to pay as your share of the cost for a medication, service or device. This can include copays, coinsurance and deductibles.
- Coverage determination- the first decision made by your drug plan about your benefits, including if the drug is covered, if you meet requirements for getting the drug, how much you must pay, whether to make an exception to a plan rule for you.

- Coverage gap- Applies to Medicare prescription drug plans - a period in which you pay higher cost sharing for prescription drugs until you spend enough to qualify for catastrophic coverage. The coverage gap, also called the donut hole, starts when you and your plan have paid a set dollar amount for medications during that year.
- Deductible- the amount you must pay for medications before your prescription drug plan begins to pay.
- Dietary supplement - a product taken orally containing one or more ingredients (such as vitamins or amino acids) intended to supplement one's diet and not considered food. These products do not have to meet safety standards of the FDA like prescription drugs or OTC's, and the claims made on the label do not have the backing of the FDA.
- Drug not covered - the drug is not on the plan's formulary. Medicare part D and most other plans typically do not cover weight loss or weight gain drugs, drugs for cosmetic purposes or hair growth, fertility drugs, drugs for sexual or erectile dysfunction, over the counter drugs, or drugs that are covered by part A or B of Medicare.
- Drug list - a list of medications covered by a prescription drug plan sometimes also called a formulary.
- Exception - a type of determination of prescription drug coverage. A formulary exception is a drug plan's decision to cover a drug that is not on its drug list or to waive a coverage rule. A tier exception is a drug plan's decision to charge a lower amount for a drug that is on its non-preferred drug tier. You or your prescriber must request an exception, and your doctor or other prescriber must provide a supporting statement explaining the medical reason for the exception.
- Extra Help- a Medicare Program to help people with limited income and resources pay their Medicare Prescription Drug Program costs, like premiums, deductibles, and coinsurance.
- Flexible spending account (FSA) - a special account you put money into that you use to pay for out of pocket health care costs. You do not pay taxes on this money. You must spend this money in a predefined amount of time (typically each plan year) or you lose the money.
- Formulary - a list of medications covered by a prescription drug plan. Also called a drug list.
- Generic drug - a prescription drug that has the same active-ingredients formula as a brand-name drug.
- Health Savings Account (HSA) - a savings account used in conjunction with a high-deductible health insurance policy that

allows users to save money tax-free against medical expenses. The money is also tax free if used on qualified medical expenses.
- Herbal supplements - Considered to be dietary supplements by the FDA and fall under the same regulations as dietary supplements.
- High Deductible Health Plan (HDHP) - a plan with a higher deductible than a traditional insurance plan. The IRS defines a HDHP as any plan with a deductible of at least $1350 for an individual or $2700 for a family. These numbers can increase yearly.
- High Deductible Medigap Policy- a type of Medigap Policy that has a high deductible but a lower premium. You must pay the deductible before the Medigap policy pays anything.
- Initial coverage limit - once you have met your deductible, you pay coinsurance for each drug until you reach your plan's out of pocket maximum which is your initial coverage limit. Medicare patients at this point have reached the donut hole.
- In-network - pharmacies and other health care providers that have agreed to provide members of a certain insurance plan with services at a discounted price.
- Medicaid - a joint federal and state program that helps with medical costs for some people with limited income and resources. Medicaid varies state to state.
- Medically necessary - Health care services or supplies needed to diagnose or treat an illness, condition, disease or symptom and meets the accepted standards of medicine.
- Medicare - Federal health insurance program for people over 65, certain people with disabilities or End stage renal disease ESRD.
- Medicare Advantage Prescription Drug Plan - a Medicare Advantage Plan that offers Medicare Prescription Drug Coverage (Part D), part A and Part B benefits all in one plan.
- Medicare Part A (hospital insurance) - Part A covers inpatient hospital stays, skilled nursing facilities, hospice care and some home health care.
- Medicare Part B (medical insurance) - Part B covers certain doctors' services, outpatient care, medical supplies, and some medications administered in a doctor's office.
- Medicare Plan - Any way other than original Medicare that you can get your Medicare health or prescription drug coverage. Term includes Medicare Prescription Drug Plans.
- Medicare Prescription Drug Coverage (Part D) - Optional benefits for prescription drugs available to all people with Medicare for an additional charge. This is offered by insurance companies and other private companies approved by Medicare.

- Medicare Savings Program - A Medicaid program that helps people with limited income and resources pay some or all of their Medicare premiums, deductibles, and coinsurance.
- Medigap policy - Medicare supplement insurance sold by private insurance companies to fill in "gaps" in original Medicare coverage.

- Network - the facilities, providers and suppliers your health insurer or plan has contracted with to provide health care services.
- Network pharmacies - Pharmacies that have agreed to provide members of a certain health plan with services at a discounted price.
- Non-preferred pharmacy - a pharmacy that's part of a drug plan's network but isn't a preferred pharmacy. You may pay higher out of pocket costs if you get your prescriptions from a non-preferred pharmacy instead of a preferred one.
- Out of network - A benefit that may be provided by your plan. Generally, this benefit gives you the choice to get plan services from outside the plan's network. In some cases, your out of pocket costs may be higher for an out of network benefit.
- Out of pocket costs - Health or prescription drug costs that you must pay on your own because they aren't covered by insurance.
- Over the Counter drugs (OTC's)- are medicines sold directly to a consumer without a prescription from a healthcare professional, as opposed to prescription drugs, which may be sold only to consumers possessing a valid prescription. The FDA still reviews data on the safety and efficacy of OTC drugs.
- Penalty - an amount added to your monthly premium for Part B or Part D if you don't join when you first become eligible. You pay this higher amount if you have Medicare.
- Pharmacy network - Pharmacies that have agreed to provide members of certain health plans with services at a discounted price. In some plans, your prescriptions are only covered if you get them filled at network pharmacies.
- Preferred pharmacy - a pharmacy that is part of a drug plan's network. You pay lower out of pocket costs if you get your prescription drugs from a preferred pharmacy instead of a non-preferred pharmacy.
- Premium - the periodic payment to Medicare, an insurance company, or a health care plan for health or prescription drug coverage.
- Preventive services - Health care to prevent illness or detect illness at an early stage, when treatment is likely to work best.
- Prior Authorization - approval that you must get from a drug plan before you fill your prescription for the prescription to be covered by your plan.
- Secondary payer - The insurance policy, plan or program that pays second on a claim for a prescription.

- State Medical Assistance (Medicaid) office - a state or local agency that can give information about and help with applications for Medicaid programs that help pay medical bills for people with limited income and resources.
- State Pharmaceutical Assistance Program (SPAP) - A state program that provides help paying for drug coverage based on financial need, age, or medical condition.
- Step Therapy - A coverage rule used by drug plans that requires you to try one or more similar, lower cost drugs to treat your condition before the plan will cover the prescribed drug.
- Tiers - Groups of drugs that have a different cost for each group. Generally, a drug in a lower tier will cost you less than a drug in a higher tier.

Appendix B: Medication List

Prescription for Maximum Savings

www.bestrxforsavings.com **Medication List as of**

Medication / Strength / Form

Date Started — Color / Shape

How I take

Reason for use

Prescriber — Pharmacy

Medication / Strength / Form

Date Started — Color / Shape

How I take

Reason for use

Prescriber — Pharmacy

Medication / Strength / Form

Date Started — Color / Shape

How I take

Reason for use

Prescriber — Pharmacy

Medication / Strength / Form

Date Started — Color / Shape

How I take

Reason for use

Prescriber — Pharmacy

Medication / Strength / Form	
Date Started	Color / Shape
How I take	
Reason for use	
Prescriber	Pharmacy

Medication / Strength / Form	
Date Started	Color / Shape
How I take	
Reason for use	
Prescriber	Pharmacy

Medication / Strength / Form	
Date Started	Color / Shape
How I take	
Reason for use	
Prescriber	Pharmacy

Medication / Strength / Form	
Date Started	Color / Shape
How I take	
Reason for use	
Prescriber	Pharmacy

Appendix C: Medication Talking Points

Medication Talking Points

BestRXforSavings.com

Current Medication:

Drug strength & form:

Started _____   Who told me to take?

Reason for use?   Helping me?

Lifestyle changes   Goal Med to stop

Side effects?   Can I D/C?

Current copay   What tier?   Other tier cost?

365 days / Days supply ⌄   = Fills/yr

Copay   x Fills/yr   = Annual Cost

Savings options:

Mail Order copay   Mail order days supply ⌄

365 days / Days supply ⌄   = Fills/yr

Mail order Copay   X Fills/yr   =Annual mail cost

Annual cost today   − Annual mail cost   =Mail Savings

Is drug generic? ⌄   Available as generic? ⌄

$4 generic exist? ⌄   Is drug Multi Source? ⌄

Prescription for Maximum Savings

Best cash/ discount price?	X Fills/yr	=Annual cash/ discount cost
Best OTC price?	X Fills/yr	=Annual OTC cost
Best Multi source price?	X Fills/yr	=Annual Multi source cost

For the best price option above, will a larger quantity cost less?

Price 90 days
Price 120 days
Price ___ days

Best large quantity price?	X Fills/yr	=Annual cost large quantity
Best half tab quantity price	X Fills/yr	=Annual half tab price

Therapeutic equivalent exist?	∨	True allergy to therapeutic equivalent?	∨
Drug 1			
Drug 2			
Drug 3			
Drug 1 price	X Fills/yr	=Annual cost drug 1	
Drug 2 price	X Fills/yr	=Annual cost drug 2	
Drug 3 price	X Fills/yr	=Annual cost drug 3	

Is this med available as a combination med with another med I take?

Drug 1

Drug 2

Combo drug cash or discount price	X Fills/yr	=Annual cash or discount cost combo drug

Jason Reed

Combo drug copay price	X Fills/yr	=Annual copay combo drug
Annual cost today	− Annual combo drugs cost	= Combo savings

Combination pill I take today that can be split into cheaper options?

Drug 1

Drug 2

Drug 1 cash price	X Fills/yr	=Annual cash cost drug 1
Drug 2 cash price	X Fills/yr	=Annual cash cost drug 2
Drug 1 copay price	X Fills/yr	=Annual copay cost drug 1
Drug 2 copay price	X Fills/yr	=Annual copay cost drug 2

Total annual cost drug 1 + drug 2 =

Annual cost today	− Annual cost of split combo	Split savings

Dosage Form

Fills saved per year	x Cost/fill	= Savings/yr

Samples Available?	☐ Yes ☐ No	How long is med trial period?
Have enough samples for trial period?	☐ Yes ☐ No	Savings from Samples

PAP, State PAP, Extra Help program(s) I am eligible for				
Do you charge to complete PAP forms?	○ Yes ○ No	If yes, what is your fee?		
Medication Coupon?	˅	How many dollars will coupon pay?		
Current annual cost		− copay savings		=New annual cost with coupon
Does my insurance have a copay coupon accumulator?	˅	Will I have to pay full deductible when coupon runs out?		˅
Am I eligible for a hardship exception from manufacturer?	˅	If yes, do you charge to complete paperwork?	☐ Yes ☐ No	
If yes, what is charge?				
Is a Biosimilar available?	˅			
What is the cost per fill?		X Fills/yr		=Annual cost
Annual cost of current drug?		− Annual cost Biosimar		=Biosimilar savings
Influenza	˅	Shingles	˅	
Pneumococcal	˅	Hepatitis B	˅	HPV ˅

About the Author

My Journey has taken me from pharmacy school at Butler University to working both retail and hospital pharmacy. My next stop was a large pharmacy benefit manager (PBM) where I had unique rolls for a pharmacist. I learned the intricacies of insurance benefits and how they collided with the clinical side of what doctors and pharmacists are trying to do for patients.

I have been on the front lines and seen the patients, family and friends who have asked the question "How am I going to pay for my medications next month?" That is not the way it has to be, but too many patients find themselves in that very situation.

Knowledge is power, and my goal is to spread the word on ways to ease the financial burden of how to pay for medications. A key part of obtaining that goal is to empower patients to confirm if a medication is really what they need.

References

1. Kesselheim AS, Avorn J, Sarpatwari A. (2016) The High Cost of Prescription Drugs in the United States: Origins and Prospects for Reform. *JAMA,* 316 (8), pp. 858-871.
2. Heath, Sara (2018). 85% of Patients Concerned about Healthcare Costs, Quality. Accessed through https://patientengagementhit.com/news/85-of-patients-concerned-about-healthcare-costs-quality
3. N. (2016). NHE Fact Sheet. Accessed through https://www.cms.gov/research-statistics-data-and-systems/statistics-trends-and-reports/nationalhealthexpenddata/nhe-fact-sheet.html
4. Sussman, Anna (2016). Burden of Healthcare Costs Moves to the Middle Class. Accessed through https://patientengagementhit.com/news/85-of-patients-concerned-about-healthcare-costs-quality
5. N. (2016). Average Annual Workplace Family Health Premiums. Accessed through www.kff.org/health-costs/press-release/average-annual-workplace-family-health-premiums-rise-modest -3-to-18142-in-2016
6. N. (2016) Quintile IMS. Accessed through https://consumer.healthday.com/general-health-information-16/prescription-drug-news-551/americans-taking-more-prescription-drugs-than-ever-survey-725208.html
7. N. (2017). Americans Taking More Prescription Drugs Than Ever: Survey. Accessed through https://consumer.healthday.com/general-health-information-16/prescription-drug-news-551/americans-taking-more-prescription-drugs-than-ever-survey-725208.html
8. Murray, Patty. (2018) Reducing Health Care Costs: Examining how Transparency Can Lower Spending and Empower Patients. Accessed through https://www.help.senate.gov/

9. Pollack, Andrew. (2015) Drug Goes From $13.50 a Tablet to $750, Overnight. Accessed through https://www.nytimes.com/2015/09/21/business/a-huge-overnight-increase-in-a-drugs-price-raises-protests.html
10. N. (2017). Pharmaceutical Industry Direct to Consumer Media Spending in the United States from 2009 to 2017 (in billion U.S. dollars). Accessed through https://www.statista.com/statistics/317819/pharmaceutical-industry-dtc-media-spending-usa/
11. Fein, Adam. (2018). Democrats and Republicans Agree: Drug Channels is Awesome! Accessed through https://www.drugchannels.net/2018/07/democrats-and-republicans-agree-drug.html#mor
12. N. (2018). Rising Drug Prices. Accessed through https://www.fiercehealthcare.com/finance/rising-drug-prices-healthc
13. N. (2018). Where Does Your Health Care Dollar Go? Accessed through https://www.ahip.org/wp-content/uploads/2017/03/HealthCareDollar_FINAL.pdf
14. Rockoff, Jonathan. (2018) This Form of Zolpidem Tartrate now Costs over 800% more. Accessed through https://www.pharmacist.com/article/form-zolpidem-tartrate-now-costs-over-800-more
15. N. (2016) NHE Fact Sheet. Accessed through https://www.cms.gov/research-statistics-data-and-systems/statistics-trends-and-reports/nationalhealthexpenddata/nhe-fact-sheet.html
16. N. (2016). Average Annual Growth Rate of Prescription Drug Spending per capita for 1960-2016. Accessed through https://www.healthsystemtracker.org/chart-collection/recent-forecasted-trends-prescription-drug-spending/#item-growth-prescription-spending-slowed-2016-increasing-rapidly-2014-2015_2016
17. N. (2017). Number of Retail Prescription Drugs Filled at Pharmacies by Payer. Accessed through http://kff.org/health-costs/state-indicator/total-retail-rx-drugs/?currentTimeframe=0&sortModel=%7B%22colId%22:%22Location%22,%22sort%22:%22asc%22%7D
18. Carr, Teresa. (2017) Too Many Meds? America's Love Affair with Prescription Medication. Accessed through https://www.consumerreports.org/prescription-drugs/too-many-meds-americas-love-affair-with-prescription-medication/
19. N. (2014). 35 FDA- Approved Prescription Drugs Later Pulled from the Market. Accessed through https://prescriptiondrugs.procon.org/view.resource.php?resourceID=005528
20. Tarn, Derjun et. al. (2006) Physician Communication When Prescribing New Medications, Archives of Internal Medicine:166:pp.1855-1862

21. N. (2018). Immunization. Accessed through http://www.who.int/topics/immunization/en/
22. N. (2017). Influenza. Accessed through http://www.nfid.org/influenza
23. Nichols, Hannah. (2017). The Top 10 Leading Causes of Death in the United States. Accessed through https://www.medicalnewstoday.com/articles/282929.php
24. N. (2016). Adult Obesity Facts. Accessed through www.cdc.gov/obesity/data/adult.html
25. Tirrell, Meg. (2018) Diabetes Defeated by Diet: How New Fresh-food Prescriptions are Beating Pricey Drugs. Accessed through https://www.cnbc.com/2018/06/20/diabetes-defeated-by-diet-new-fresh-food-prescriptions-beat-drugs.html
26. N. (2014). The Health Consequences of Smoking. Accessed through https://www.surgeongeneral.gov/library/reports/50-years-of-progress/index.html
27. N. (2018). The Framingham Heart Study. Accessed through https://www.framinghamheartstudy.org/
28. N. (2016). How is the Body Affected by Sleep Deprivation? Accessed through https://www.nichd.nih.gov/health/topics/sleep/conditioninfo/Pages/sleep-deprivation.aspx#f6
29. Altavela, JL. (2010). The Epidemiology of Prescriptions Abandoned at the Pharmacy. Accessed through https://www.ncbi.nlm.nih.gov/pubmed/21576546
30. N. (2017). QuickFacts United States. Accessed through https://www.census.gov/quickfacts/fact/table/US/PST045217
31. N. (2013). Analyzing 9.5 Million Part D Prescription Claims. Accessed through https://money.cnn.com/2018/06/03/news/economy/medicare-drugs-cash-price/index.html
32. N. (2017) Shop Around for Better Drug Prices. Accessed through www.consumerreports.org/durg-prices/shop-around-for-better-drug-prices/
33. N. (2014). JNC 8 Hypertension Guideline Algorithm. Accessed through http://www.nmhs.net/documents/27JNC8HTNGuidelinesBookBooklet.pdf
34. N. (2016). Drug for Depression. Accessed through https://secure.medicalletter.org/article-share?a=1498b&p=tml&title=Drugs%20for%20Depression&cannotaccesstitle=1
35. Sacks, Chana. (2016). Medicare Spending on Brand Name Combination Medications vs their Generic Constituents. Accessed through https://jamanetwork.com/journals/jama/article-abstract/2697695
36. N. (2006). Consumers Often Overdose on Prescription Eye Drops. Accessed through https://www.consumeraffairs.com/news04/2006/09/pubcit_eye_drops.html

37. N. (2006). No More Free Drug Samples? Accessed throughhttps://www.ncbi.nlm.nih.gov/pmc/articles/PMC2669216/
38. N. (2017). One Million Medicare Part D Enrollees Had Out of Pocket Drug Costs Above the Catastrophic Threshold in 2015. Accessed through https://www.kff.org/medicare/press-release/one-million-medicare-part-d-enrollees-had-out-of-pocket-drug-costs-above-the-catastrophic-threshold-in-2015/
39. N. (2017). Share of Total Patient Out-of-Pocket by Cost Sharing Type. Accessed from IQVIA Rx Benefit Design: IQVIA Analysis.
40. N. (2017). Large U.S. Employers Project Health Care Benefit Costs to Surpass $14,000 per Employee in 2018. Accessed through https://www.businessgrouphealth.org/news/nbgh-news/press-releases/press-release-details/?ID=334
41. N. (2018). In the Driver's Seat: Accelerated Rx Rebates to Consumers. Accessed through https://www.xcenda.com/hpw-archive/health-policy-weekly-03-09-18
42. N. (2017). The Consultant Pharmacist. Accessed through https://cdn.ymaws.com/www.ascp.com/resource/resmgr/docs/TCP/2017ASCPMediaKit_FINAL.pdf
43. N. (2018). IQVIA, National Sales Perspective. Accessed through https://www.iqvia.com/locations/united-states/commercial-operations/essential-information/sales-information
44. Cohen HP, Blauvelt A, Rifkin RM, et al. Switching Reference Medicines to Biosimilars: a Systematic Literature Review of Clinical Outcomes. Drugs. 2018;78:pp 463–78
45. Miller S (2013). The $250 Billion Potential of Biosimilars. Express Scripts website. Available through http://lab.express-scripts.com/lab/insights/industry-updates/the-$250
46. Kamal, Rabah, Cox, Cynthia. (2017). What are the Recent and Forecasted Trends in Prescription Drug Spending. Accessed through https://www.healthsystemtracker.org/chart-collection/recent-forecasted-trends-prescription-drug-spending/#item-growth-prescription-spending-slowed-2016-increasing-rapidly-2014-2015_2016

Jason Reed

www.ingramcontent.com/pod-product-compliance
Lightning Source LLC
Chambersburg PA
CBHW031419210526
45464CB00005B/1960